Pharmacology

PreTest®
Self-Assessment
and Review

• NOTICE •

Pharmacology

PreTest®
Self-Assessment and Review

Seventh Edition

Senior Editor

Joseph R. DiPalma, M.D., D.Sc.
Emeritus Professor of Pharmacology and Medicine
Hahnemann University School of Medicine
Philadelphia, PA

Contributing Editors

Edward J. Barbieri, Ph.D.
Associate Professor of Pharmacology
Hahnemann University School of Medicine
Philadelphia, PA

G. John DiGregorio, M.D., Ph.D.
Professor of Pharmacology and Medicine
Hahnemann University School of Medicine
Philadelphia, PA

Andrew P. Ferko, Ph.D.
Associate Professor of Pharmacology
Hahnemann University School of Medicine
Philadelphia, PA

McGraw-Hill, Inc.
Health Professions Division/PreTest Series

New York St. Louis San Francisco Auckland
Bogotá Caracas Lisbon London Madrid
Mexico Milan Montreal New Delhi Paris
San Juan Singapore Sydney Tokyo Toronto

Pharmacology: PreTest® Self-Assessment and Review, Seventh Edition
International Editions 1993.

2 3 4 5 6 7 8 9 0 SEP 9 8 7 6 5 4 3

The editors were Gail Gavert and Bruce MacGregor.
The production supervisor was Gyl Favours.
This book was set in Times Roman by Compset, Inc.

Library of Congress Cataloging-in-Publication Data

Pharmacology : PreTest self-assessment and review / senior editor, Joseph R. DiPalma ; contributing editors, Edward J. Barbieri . . . [et al.]. - 7th ed.
Includes bibliographical references.
ISBN 0-07-051998-6
1. Pharmacology - Examinations, questions, etc.
I. DiPalma, Joseph R.
[DNLM : 1. Pharmacology - examination questions. QV18 P5365]
RM 301.13.P475 1993
615'.1'076 - dc20
DNLM/DLC
for Library of Congress 91-35343
CIP

When ordering this title, use ISBN 0-07-112781-X

Printed in Singapore

Contents

Introduction

This seventh edition of *Pharmacology: PreTest® Self-Assessment and Review* has been extensively revised to conform with recent changes in policy of the National Board of Medical Examiners. Of particular interest to takers of Step 1 of the United States Medical Licensing Examination (USMLE) is that only two types of questions will be used because all K-type (multiple true-false) questions have been eliminated. The remaining types are the one best answer items and matching sets. This simplification emphasizes memory somewhat more, but relationships and interpretations of mechanisms are still extremely important. Since only one examination qualifies as a licensing test (the Federation Licensing Examination and the Foreign Medical Graduate Examination in the Medical Sciences will probably be eliminated), some pooling of questions from these other examinations is expected. One should not anticipate that this will make the National Board examination easier; however, the questions may have a more clinical flavor.

The format of the Pretest remains essentially the same. Each question is accompanied by an answer, a paragraph of explanation, and a specific reference to a standard textbook. Sections on gastrointestinal drugs and immunology have been added. Before each chapter, a list of key terms or classifications of drugs or both is included to aid review. In addition, suggestions for effective study and review have been added below.

The most effective method of using this book is to complete one chapter at a time. Prepare yourself for each chapter by reviewing from your notes and favorite text the drugs listed at the beginning of each section. You should concentrate especially on the prototype drugs, which are marked by an asterisk. Then proceed to indicate your answer by each question, allowing yourself not more than one minute for each question. In this way you will be approximating the time limits imposed by the actual board examination.

When you finish answering the questions in a chapter, you should then spend as much time as you need verifying your answers and carefully reading the explanations. Although you should pay special attention to the explanations of questions you answered incorrectly or were uncertain about, you should read *every* explanation to reinforce your memory. The contributors to this work have designed the explanations to expand and supplement the information tested by the questions. If, after reading the explanation for an answer, you feel you need still more information about the material covered, you should consult the references indicated.

SUGGESTIONS FOR EFFECTIVE STUDY AND REVIEW

The study of pharmacology is not different from that of the other basic medical sciences. For most students it has more relevance to clinical medicine than do biochemistry or anatomy. It has the advantage of coming last in the curriculum of basic sciences. Nevertheless, the disadvantage of pharmacology is the need to commit to memory an enormous number of names and facts about numerous drugs and furthermore to relate these to each other and to clinical medicine. Most students find it advantageous to learn a classification of drugs that enables them to immediately place a drug into a category that characterizes the likely pharmacology. In addition the main or original drug in each category (the prototype drug) should be thoroughly studied. The close relatives need merely to be known by name and with reference to their advantages over the prototype drug.

Though it may be obvious, it is still worth repeating that a minimum knowledge of prototype drugs consists of the following:

1. *Chemistry.* You should be able to recognize the structural formula. Are there any structure-activity relationships (SARs)? What is the main ring structure? steroid? quinoline? benzodiazepine? sympathetic amine? etc.

2. *Mechanism of Action.* This usually consists of two parts: (1) molecular and (2) cellular or physiologic. Mechanisms of action mainly explain pharmacodynamics or effects on organ systems that are of most use in a clinical knowledge of the drug. For example, does the drug lower blood pressure and, if so, does it do so by vasodilation, negative inotropic effects on the heart, central nervous system mechanisms, etc.?

3, *Pharmacokinetics.* This covers absorption, distribution, and elimination of the drug. What is the usual route of administration of the drug? What is its half-life, degree of protein binding, etc.? *The dose of the drug is usually not asked in modern examinations.*

4. *Clinical Use.* You should know FDA indications plus medically accepted uses.

5. *Toxicity.* This includes adverse reactions and serious toxicities, such as nephritis, hepatitis, blood dyscrasia, etc. You should know important drug interactions.

With respect to names of drugs, the generic name must be known even though the trade name is often more commonly used. In this text, the generic name is always used and often, especially when it is a relatively new drug, the trade name is mentioned as well. It is advantageous to memorize certain endings because they give a clue as to the category in which a drug belongs. The following are examples of endings of generic names:

Ending	Drug
-olol	**beta blockers**
-cillin	**penicillin-type antibiotic**
-azine	**phenothiazine-type antipsychotic**
-epam	**benzodiazepine-type CNS drugs**
-azide	**thiazide-like diuretics**
-cline	**tetracycline-type antibiotics**

Ending	Drug
-mycin	miscellaneous antibiotics
-opril	angiotensin converting enzyme inhibitors
-bital	barbiturate sedative-hypnotic
-idine	histamine H_2 antagonist

General Principles

Drug-Receptor Interaction
- Dose-response relationship
  - Graded dose-response curve
  - Quantal dose-response curve
  - Time-action curves
  - Therapeutic index
  - Drug assays, biologic vs chemical
- Receptors
  - Nature of the drug-receptor interaction
  - Structure and activity relationship (SAR)
  - Physical chemistry of the drug-receptor association
  - Relationship to Michaelis-Menten enzyme kinetics
- Simultaneous action of two drugs
  - Additive effects
  - Potentiation
  - Synergism
  - Competitive antagonism
  - Noncompetitive antagonism
- Other factors in drug-receptor interaction
  - Tolerance
  - Tachyphylaxis
  - Up and down regulation by the number of receptors
  - Scatchard plot

Molecular Models of Receptors and Transduction Mechanisms
1. Ion channel receptors
   - Nicotine
   - GABA
   - Glycine
   - Gutamate (NMDA, quisqualate, kainate)
   - Transduction mechanism = ionic
2. Receptor–G protein–effector system
   - Beta adrenergic
   - Muscarinic
   - Serotonin
   - Angiotensin
   - Rhodopsin
   - Transduction mechanism = G protein linked by guanine diphosphate and triphosphate (GDP-GTP) linked to adenylate-cyclase activity, phospholipase, potassium, and calcium channels
3. Receptor tyrosine kinases
   - Erythrocyte growth factor (EGF)
   - Platelet-derived growth factor (PDGF)
   - Insulin
   - Transduction mechanism = Activation of protein kinases
4. Steroid hormone receptors
   - Thyroid hormone
   - Vitamin D
   - Estrogen
   - Progesterone
   - Glucocorticoid
   - Transduction mechanism = transcriptional changes by binding to DNA

Biotransformation
- Lipophilic versus hydrophilic considerations
- Phase I reactions
  - Oxidations
  - Reductions
  - Hydrolysis
  - Effect on water solubility

- Phase II reactions
  - Conjugations
    - Glucuronic acid
    - Glutathione
    - Sulfate
  - Effect on water solubility
- Microsomal cytochrome P-450
  - Oxidation reactions
    - Aliphatic and aromatic hydroxylations
    - Epioxidation
    - N, O, and S dealkylation
    - Sulfoxidation
    - Desulfuration
    - Dehalogenation
- Nonmicrosomal oxidations
  - Alcohol
  - Aldehyde
  - Monoamine
  - Diamine
  - Purine
- Reduction reactions
  - Microsomal
    - Nitro, azo, dehalogenation
  - Nonmicrosomal
    - Aldehyde, ketone, quinine
- Pharmacogenetic variants
  - Slow acetylators
  - Idiosyncratic reactions to drugs

Pharmacokinetics

- Types of absorption
  - Passive transport
  - Specialized transport
- Sites of absorption
  - Alimentary canal
  - Oral mucosa
  - Rectal mucosa
  - Skin
- Routes of administration
  - Parenteral
    - Intravenous
    - Intramuscular
    - Subcutaneous
  - Respiratory tract
    - Aerosols
  - Topical
- Distribution
  - Lipid/water partition coefficient
  - Plasma protein binding
  - Tissue protein binding
- Redistribution
- Elimination
  - Renal excretion
  - Biotransformation
  - Biliary excretion
  - Minor in saliva, sweat, milk
- Pharmacokinetic models and compartments
  - One compartment
  - Two compartments
- Kinetics
  - First order

    $$\text{Slope} = \frac{-k}{2.303}$$

    Half-life ($t\frac{1}{2}$)

    $$t\tfrac{1}{2} = \frac{0.693}{k}$$
- Zero-order rate equation
- Volume of distribution (V_d)

  $$V_d = \frac{\text{Total amount of drug in the body}}{\text{concentration of drug in plasma}}$$
- Distribution phase vs elimination phase determined in plasma concentration × time curves
- Clearance

  $$CL_{total} = V_d \times k_e = \frac{0.693 \times V_d}{t\frac{1}{2}}$$

  $$t\tfrac{1}{2} = \frac{0.693 \times V_d}{CL_{total}}$$
- Dosage regimens and pharmacokinetic profiles
  - Single doses
    - Intravenous
    - Oral
  - Bioavailability
  - Multiple doses
    - Interval between doses and accumulation
  - Continuous IV infusion
  - Multiple oral dosing

- Clinical Pharmacology
  - Definition and scope
  - Statistical and epidemiologic approaches
  - Bioavailability and bioequivalence
  - Placebo effect
- Drug Interactions
  - Mechanisms
    - Enzyme stimulation (induction)
    - Enzyme inhibition
    - Gastrointestinal absorption changes
    - Protein binding
    - Adrenergic mechanisms
    - Cholinergic mechanisms
    - Neuromuscular junction
    - Drug biotransformation
    - Renal tubular transport
    - Urinary pH and drug excretion
- Factors Affecting Drug Dosage
  - Age, sex, and weight
  - Pregnancy and lactation
  - Renal disease
  - Hepatic disease
  - Pharmacogenetics
- Development of New Drugs
  - Animal vs human doses
  - Single-dose methodology
  - Open studies
  - Blind and double-blind studies
- Regulation by the Food and Drug Administration
  - Investigational new drug (IND)
  - New drug application (NDA)
  - Phase I, II, III, and IV studies
  - Postmarketing surveillance
- Ethics of Human Investigation
  - Institutional Review Board (IRB)
- Fate of marketed drugs

DIRECTIONS: Each question below contains five suggested responses. Select the **one best** response to each question.

1. All the following characteristics are associated with the process of facilitated diffusion of drugs EXCEPT

(A) the transport mechanism becomes saturated at high drug concentrations
(B) the process is selective for certain ionic or structural configurations of the drug
(C) if two compounds are transported by the same mechanism, one will competitively inhibit the transport of the other
(D) the drug crosses the membrane against a concentration gradient and the process requires cellular energy
(E) the transport process can be inhibited noncompetitively by substances that interfere with cellular metabolism

2. Which route of administration is most likely to subject a drug to a first-pass effect?

(A) Intravenous
(B) Inhalational
(C) Oral
(D) Sublingual
(E) Intramuscular

3. Drugs may be released slowly from various drug reservoirs over long periods of time. The body reservoir that holds the largest amount of the barbiturate thiopental (Pentothal) is

(A) fat
(B) lung
(C) liver
(D) muscle
(E) serum albumin

4. A 37-year-old man with pneumonia is being treated with a new penicillin derivative that is partly metabolized and partly excreted unchanged in the urine. Immediately after an initial dose of 100 mg IV, the maximum drug concentration in the plasma was measured at 10 mg/L and the elimination half-life from the patient was estimated to equal 7 h. The plasma clearance of the parent drug appearing in the urine was 8.25 mL/min. What percentage of drug elimination can be attributed to the metabolism of the compound?

(A) 10
(B) 25
(C) 50
(D) 75
(E) 90

5. The route of excretion for drugs or their metabolic derivatives that is quantitatively the LEAST significant is which of the following?

(A) Biliary tract
(B) Kidneys
(C) Lungs
(D) Feces
(E) Milk

6. If a drug is repeatedly administered at dosing intervals equal to its elimination half-life, the number of doses required for the plasma concentration of the drug to reach the steady state is

(A) 2 to 3
(B) 4 to 5
(C) 6 to 7
(D) 8 to 9
(E) 10 or more

7. The following pharmacokinetic data were obtained from a 70-kg patient treated with theophylline: plasma concentration = 10 μg/mL immediately after a dose of 5 mg/kg IV; plasma protein binding = 56 percent; biologic $t_{1/2}$ = 8 h. The total body clearance of theophylline in this patient was

(A) 1.3 L/h
(B) 3 L/h
(C) 35 L/h
(D) 43 L/h
(E) 212 L/h

8. When two pharmacologically active agents interact, the response elicited by the combination of drugs may be equal to, greater than, or less than the sum of the effects of the individual compounds. A *synergistic* effect is one in which

(A) one drug alters the pharmacokinetics of the second drug so that less of the second compound reaches the target tissue
(B) the combined effect of the two drugs is greater than the sum of the effect of each compound given alone
(C) an increased effect of one drug occurs in the presence of a compound that does not cause that effect
(D) the combined effect of the two drugs is equal to the sum of the effect of each compound given alone
(E) two drugs produce opposite effects on the same physiologic function

9. The pharmacokinetic value that most reliably reflects the amount of drug reaching the target tissue after oral administration is the

(A) peak blood concentration
(B) time to peak blood concentration
(C) product of the volume of distribution and the first-order rate constant
(D) volume of distribution
(E) area under the blood concentration–time curve

Questions 10–13

Cimetidine (Tagamet) 200 mg was administered intravenously to a 70-kg man with peptic ulcer disease. The plasma concentrations of the drug were determined at various times after injection, as shown in the figure below.

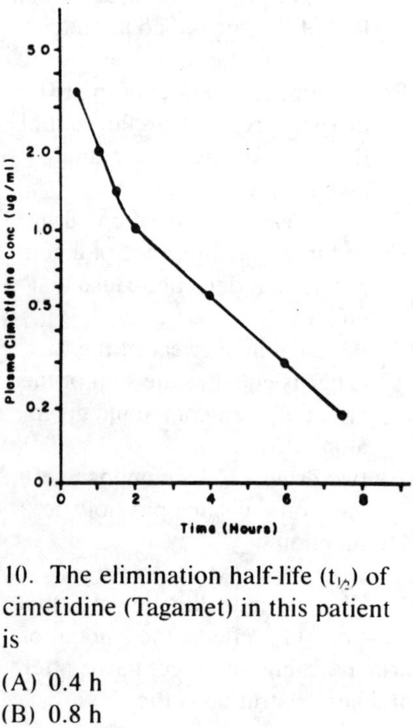

10. The elimination half-life ($t_{1/2}$) of cimetidine (Tagamet) in this patient is

(A) 0.4 h
(B) 0.8 h
(C) 1.5 h
(D) 2.3 h
(E) 4.0 h

11. The elimination rate constant (k_e) of cimetidine (Tagamet) in this patient is

(A) 0.1 h^{-1}
(B) 0.2 h^{-1}
(C) 0.3 h^{-1}
(D) 0.4 h^{-1}
(E) 0.5 h^{-1}

12. The apparent volume of distribution of cimetidine (Tagamet) in this patient is

(A) 1.6 L
(B) 39 L
(C) 59 L
(D) 111 L
(E) 200 L

13. The total body clearance of the drug is

(A) 33.5 L/h
(B) 48.0 L/h
(C) 60.0 L/h
(D) 255.0 L/h
(E) 370.5 L/h

14. All the following are phase I biotransformation reactions EXCEPT

(A) sulfoxide formation
(B) nitro reduction
(C) ester hydrolysis
(D) sulfate conjugation
(E) deamination

15. It was determined that 95 percent of an oral 80-mg dose of verapamil (Calan, Isoptin) was absorbed in a 70-kg test subject. However, because of extensive biotransformation during its first pass through the portal circulation, the bioavailability of verapamil was only 25 percent. Assuming a liver blood flow of 1500 mL/min, the hepatic clearance of verapamil in this situation was

(A) 60 mL/min
(B) 375 mL/min
(C) 740 mL/min
(D) 1110 mL/min
(E) 1425 mL/min

16. Drug products have many types of names. Of the following types of names that are applied to drugs, the one that is the official name and refers only to that drug and not to a particular product is the

(A) generic name
(B) trade name
(C) brand name
(D) chemical name
(E) proprietary name

17. An enteric-coated dosage form can be used to avoid all the following problems possible from oral drug administration EXCEPT

(A) irritation to the gastric mucosa with nausea and vomiting
(B) destruction of the drug by gastric acid or digestive enzymes
(C) unpleasant taste of the drug
(D) formation of nonabsorbable drug-food complexes
(E) variability in absorption caused by fluctuations in gastric emptying time

18. Which of the following is classified as belonging to the tyrosine kinase family of receptors?

(A) $GABA_A$ receptor
(B) β-Adrenergic receptor
(C) Insulin receptor
(D) Nicotinic-II receptor
(E) Hydrocortisone receptor

19. All the following statements concerning binding of drugs to plasma proteins are true EXCEPT

(A) acidic drugs generally bind to plasma albumin; basic drugs preferentially bind to α_1-acidic glycoprotein
(B) plasma protein binding is a reversible process
(C) binding sites on plasma proteins are nonselective and drugs with similar physicochemical characteristics compete for these limited sites
(D) the fraction of the drug in the plasma that is bound is inactive and generally unavailable for systemic distribution
(E) plasma protein binding generally limits renal tubular secretion and biotransformation

20. All the following compounds are prodrugs that are biotransformed to a pharmacologically active product EXCEPT

(A) minoxidil (Loniten)
(B) enalapril maleate (Vasotec)
(C) diazepam (Valium)
(D) sulfasalazine (Azulfidine)
(E) sulindac (Clinoril)

21. The figure below shows the change in mean blood pressure as a result of increasing doses of norepinephrine and the antagonism of this response by drugs X and Y. Using the information provided in the diagram, which statement is correct?

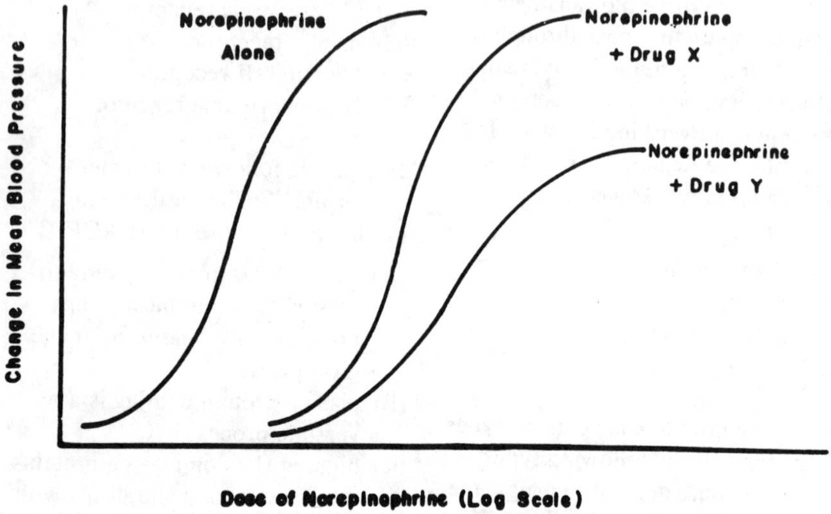

(A) Drug X is a more potent antagonist than drug Y
(B) Drug X is a more effective antagonist than drug Y
(C) Drug Y shows the characteristics of competitive antagonism
(D) Drug Y shows the characteristics of noncompetitive antagonism
(E) None of the above

22. The greater proportion of the dose of a drug administered orally will be absorbed in the small intestine. However, on the assumption that passive transport of the nonionized form of a drug determines its rate of absorption, which of the following compounds will be absorbed to the LEAST extent in the stomach?

(A) Ampicillin (pK_a = 2.5)
(B) Aspirin (pK_a = 3.0)
(C) Warfarin (pK_a = 5.0)
(D) Phenobarbital (pK_a = 7.4)
(E) Propranolol (pK_a = 9.4)

DIRECTIONS: Each group of questions below consists of lettered headings followed by a set of numbered items. For each numbered item select the **one** lettered heading with which it is **most** closely associated. Each lettered heading may be used **once, more than once, or not at all.**

Questions 23–25

For each type of drug interaction below, select the pair of substances that illustrates it with a *reduction* in drug effectiveness.

(A) Tetracycline and milk
(B) Amobarbital (Amytal) and secobarbital (Seconal)
(C) Isoproterenol (Isuprel) and propranolol (Inderal)
(D) Soap and benzalkonium chloride (Ionil)
(E) Sulfamethoxazole and trimethoprim

23. Therapeutic interaction

24. Physical interaction

25. Chemical interaction

Questions 26–28

For each description of a drug response below, choose the term with which it is most likely to be associated.

(A) Supersensitivity
(B) Tachyphylaxis
(C) Tolerance
(D) Hyposensitivity
(E) Anaphylaxis

26. Immunologically mediated reaction to drug observed soon after administration

27. A rapid reduction in the effect of a given dose of a drug after only one or two doses

28. Hyperreactivity to a drug seen as a result of denervation

Questions 29–33

Many families of drugs consist of members that vary only with respect to substituents on a common ring structure. For each type of pharmacologic effect that follows, select the ring structure with which it is most likely to be associated.

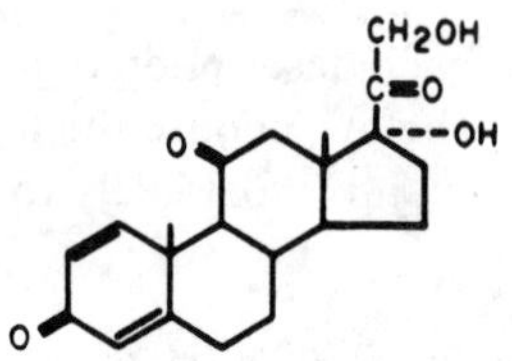

A

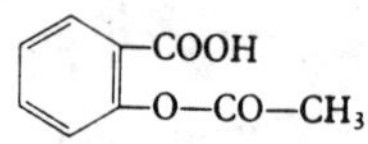

B

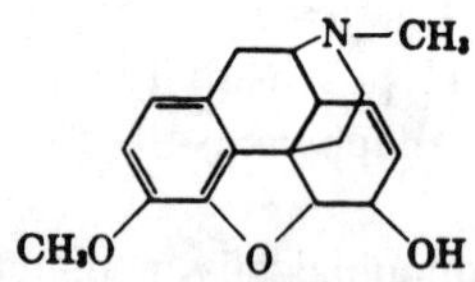

C

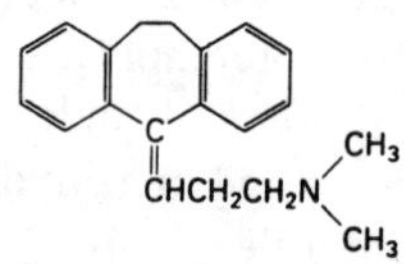

D

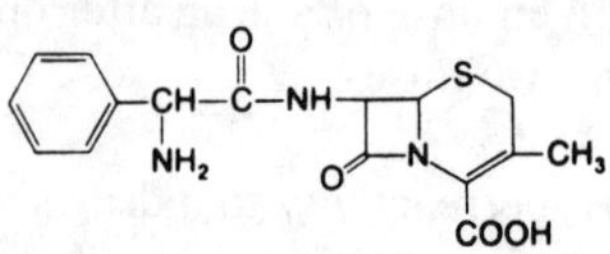

E

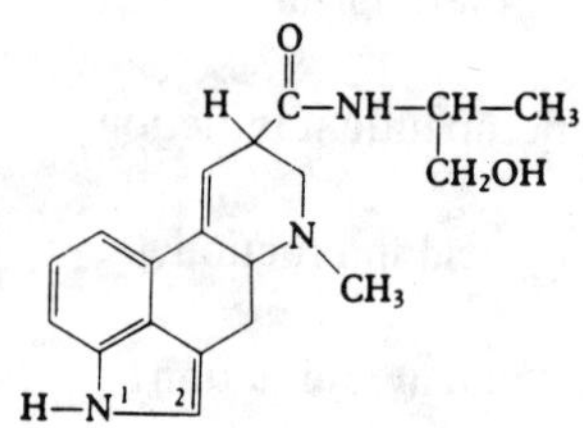

F

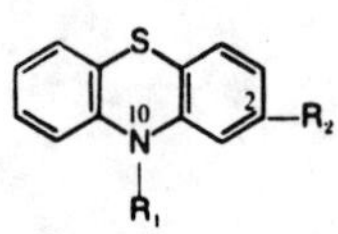

G

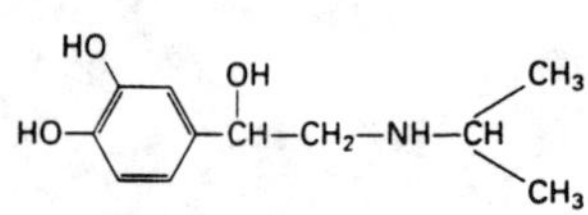

H

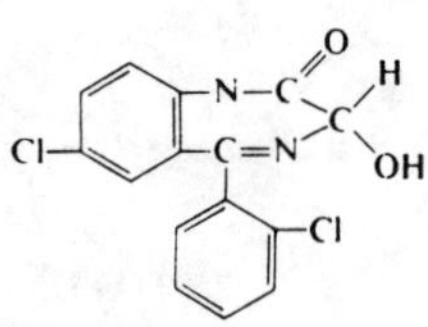

I

29. Bronchodilator

30. Opioid analgesic

31. Antipsychotic

32. Antimicrobial

33. Corticosteroid anti-inflammatory

Questions 34–36

For each component of a time-action curve listed below, choose the lettered interval (shown on the diagram) with which it is most closely associated.

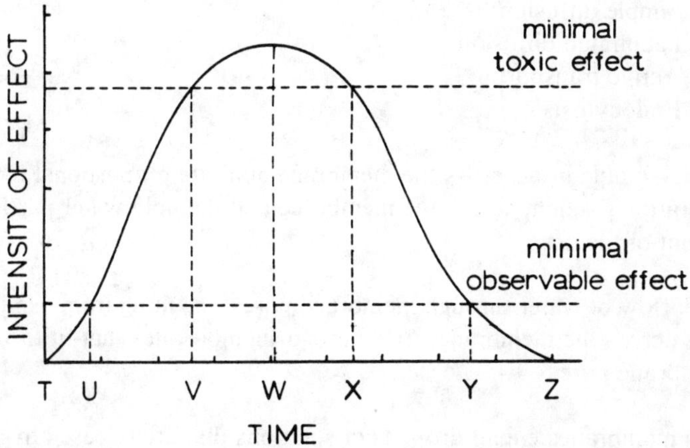

(A) T to U
(B) T to V
(C) T to W
(D) T to Z
(E) U to V
(F) U to W
(G) U to X
(H) U to Y
(I) V to X
(J) X to Y

34. Time to peak effect

35. Time to onset of action

36. Duration of action

Questions 37–39

For each description below, select the transmembranal transport mechanism it best defines.

(A) Filtration
(B) Simple diffusion
(C) Facilitated diffusion
(D) Active transport
(E) Endocytosis

37. Lipid-soluble drugs cross the membrane at a rate proportional to the concentration gradient across the membrane and the lipid:water partition coefficient of the drug

38. Bulk flow of water through membrane pores, resulting from osmotic differences across the membrane, transports drug molecules that fit through the membrane pores

39. Cell membranes engulf droplets of solutions that are released inside the cell

Questions 40–42

Lipid-soluble xenobiotics are commonly biotransformed by oxidation in the drug-metabolizing microsomal system (DMMS). For each description below, choose the component of the microsomal mixed-function oxidase system with which it is most closely associated.

(A) NADPH
(B) Cytochrome *a*
(C) ATP
(D) NADPH–cytochrome P-450 reductase
(E) Monoamine oxidase
(F) Cyclooxygenase
(G) Cytochrome P-450

40. A group of iron-containing isoenzymes that activate molecular oxygen to a form capable of interacting with organic substrates

41. The component that provides reducing equivalents for the enzyme system

42. A flavoprotein that accepts reducing equivalents and transfers them to the catalytic enzyme

General Principles
Answers

1. **The answer is D.** *(DiPalma, 3/e. pp 34–35.)* Drugs can be transferred across biologic membranes by passive processes (i.e., filtration and simple diffusion) and by specialized processes (i.e., active transport, facilitated diffusion, and pinocytosis). Active transport is a carrier-mediated process that shows all the characteristics listed in the question. Facilitated diffusion is similar to active transport except that the drug is *not* transported against a concentration gradient and *no* energy is required for this carrier-mediated system to function. Pinocytosis usually involves transport of proteins and macromolecules by a complex process in which a cell engulfs the compound within a membrane-bound vesicle.

2. **The answer is C.** *(DiPalma, 3/e. pp 37–38, 49. Gilman, 8/e. p 5.)* The first-pass effect is commonly considered to involve the biotransformation of a drug during its first passage through the portal circulation of the liver. Drugs that are administered orally and rectally enter the portal circulation of the liver and can be biotransformed by this organ prior to reaching the systemic circulation. Therefore, drugs with a *high* first-pass effect are highly biotransformed quickly, which reduces the oral bioavailability and the systemic blood concentrations of the compounds. Administration by the intravenous, intramuscular, and sublingual routes allows the drug to attain concentrations in the systemic circulation and to be distributed throughout the body prior to hepatic metabolism. In most cases, drugs administered by inhalation are not subjected to a significant first-pass effect unless the respiratory tissue is a major site for the drug's biotransformation.

3. **The answer is A.** *(DiPalma, 3/e. pp 41, 42. Gilman, 8/e. p 12.)* Body fat may contain up to 70 percent of an administered dose of lipid-soluble thiopental 3 h after injection. Other drugs may tend to accumulate in muscle or liver. For example, the concentration of the antimalarial drug quinacrine can be one thousand times greater in liver than in plasma. Serum albumin binds many drugs, some to appreciable degrees, thus reducing the free fraction that is pharmacologically effective. Plasma-bound drugs are readily released as the effective components are consumed by biotransfusion or excretion. Drugs are usually released much more slowly from fat because fat has a relatively limited blood supply.

4. The answer is C. *(DiPalma, 3/e. pp 48–49. Gilman, 8/e. pp 22–25.)* The total body clearance (CL_{total}) can be calculated by the equation

$$CL_{total} = \frac{(0.693)\,(V_d)}{t_{1/2}}$$

where V_d is the apparent volume of distribution and $t_{1/2}$ is the half-life. V_d = 10 L (100 mg dose/10 mg/L plasma concentration). Therefore,

$$CL_{total} = \frac{(0.693)\,(10\text{ L})}{7\text{ h}}$$

$$CL_{total} = 0.99\text{ L/h or }16.5\text{ mL/min}$$

CL_{total} represents the sum of clearance from all participating organs in the body, but mainly liver and kidney; that is,

$$CL_{total} = CL_{liver} + CL_{kidney}$$

Since clearance of the parent drug in the urine (unmetabolized) was 8.25 mL/min, this occurred via the kidney. Therefore,

$$CL_{total} - CL_{kidney} = CL_{liver}$$

$$16.50\text{ mL/min} - 8.25\text{ mL/min} = 8.25\text{ mL/min}$$

or 50 percent of drug elimination is attributed to metabolism.

5. The answer is E. *(DiPalma, 3/e. pp 41–43. Gilman, 8/e. pp 18–20.)* The amounts of drugs excreted in milk are small compared with those excreted by other routes; but drugs in milk may have significant, undesired pharmacologic effects on breast-fed infants. The principal route of excretion of the products of a given drug varies with the drug. Some drugs are predominantly excreted by the kidneys, whereas others leave the body in the bile and feces. Inhalation anesthetic agents are eliminated by the lungs. The path of excretion may affect the clinical choice of a drug, as is the case with renal failure or hepatic insufficiency.

6. The answer is B. *(Gilman, 8/e. pp 26–27. Katzung, 4/e. pp 36–37.)* When a drug is administered in multiple doses and each dose is given prior to the complete elimination of the previous dose, the mean plasma concentration ($\bar{C}$) of the drug during each dose interval rises as shown in the following figure:

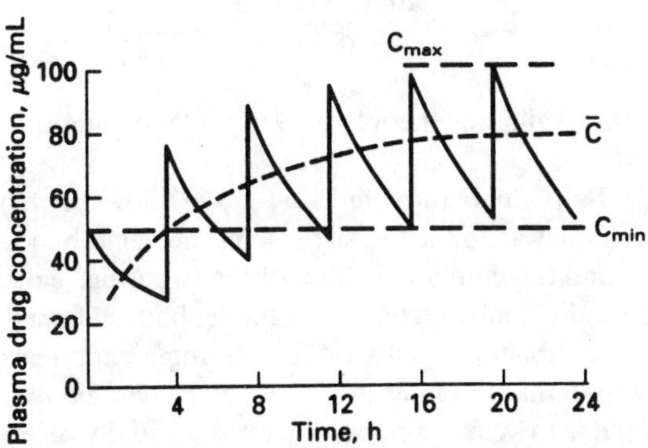

(From DiPalma and DiGregorio, with permission.)

The plasma concentration will continue to rise until it reaches a plateau, or steady state. At this time, the plasma concentration will fluctuate between a maximum (C_{max}) and a minimum (C_{min}) level, but, more importantly, the amount of drug eliminated per dose interval will equal the amount of drug absorbed per dose. When a drug is given at a dosing interval equal to its elimination half-life, it will reach 50 percent of its steady state plasma concentration after one half-life, 75 percent after two half-lives, 87.5 percent after three, 93.75 percent after four, and 96.87 percent after five. Thus, from a practical viewpoint, regardless of the magnitude of the dose or the half-life, the steady state will be achieved in four to five half-lives.

7. The answer is B. *(DiPalma, 3/e. pp 48–49. Katzung, 4/e. pp 32–33.)* Total body clearance is defined as the rate of removal of a drug from the body. It is the sum of the individual clearance rates provided by the kidney, liver, lung, saliva, milk, and so on and is calculated according to the equation

$$CL_{total} = \frac{0.693\ V_d}{t_{1/2}}$$

where CL_{total} is the total body clearance in liters per hour, V_d is the apparent volume of distribution in liters, and $t_{1/2}$ is the biologic half-life in hours. The V_d is found by dividing the total amount of drug in the body (5 mg/kg IV, 70 kg = 350 mg) by the plasma concentration at time zero (10 μg/mL), and in this problem it equals 35 L. After substitution of the appropriate values into the equation above, the answer is calculated

$$CL_{total} = \frac{(0.693)\ (35\ L)}{(8\ h)} = 3\ L/h$$

which is the average value for theophylline expected in adults.

8. The answer is B. *(Gilman, 8/e. pp 53–54.) Synergism* refers to a situation in which two drugs act at the same site, or on the same biologic unit (cell, tissue, or organ), and the combined effect of the two drugs exceeds the algebraic sum of their individual effects. For example, both sulfamethoxazole and trimethoprim have antibacterial activity, but the combination has greater bactericidal activity than that of either drug used alone. *Potentiation* (described in choice C) is similar to synergism, but the term is usually reserved for cases in which two drugs act differently, one drug having no significant effect alone. For example, isopropyl alcohol is not hepatotoxic, but it greatly enhances the liver toxicity produced by carbon tetrachloride. An *additive effect* (described in choice D) occurs when the combined effect of two drugs acting by the same mechanism is equal to that expected by simple addition.

Antagonism is the interference of one drug with the action of another. *Pharmacologic antagonism* is the interaction that occurs through receptor-mediated events; e.g., atropine blocks the effects of acetylcholine at muscarinic receptor sites. *Dispositional antagonism* (described in choice A) is an alteration in the absorption, distribution, biotransformation, or excretion of a compound so that less compound can reach the active site; e.g., chronic administration of phenobarbital enhances the metabolism of many drugs through the hepatic drug microsomal metabolizing system and reduces their effects. *Functional,* or *physiologic, antagonism* (choice E) is observed when two compounds produce opposite effects on the same system; e.g., histamine-induced bronchoconstriction is antagonized by epinephrine, a bronchodilator. *Chemical antagonism* results from a chemical interaction between compounds that neutralizes their effects; e.g., deferoxamine chelates with iron and reduces its concentrations throughout the body.

9. The answer is E. *(Gilman, 8/e. p 25.)* The fraction of a drug dose absorbed after oral administration is affected by a wide variety of factors that can strongly influence the peak blood levels and the time to peak blood concentration. The volume of distribution and the total body clearance (volume of distribution × first-order elimination rate constant) also are important in determining the amount of drug that reaches the target tissue. Only the area under the blood concentration–time curve, however, reflects absorption, distribution, metabolism, and excretion factors; it is the most reliable and popular method of evaluating bioavailability.

10. The answer is D. *(DiPalma, 3/e. pp 44–47.)* The figure shows an elimination pattern that has two components. The upper linear portion represents distribution of cimetidine from the plasma to the tissues and is the alpha phase of elimination. True elimination is represented by the lower linear portion of the line (the beta phase), and this is what is used to determine the elimination half-life of the drug. This pattern typifies a two-compartment model. At 2 h after administration, the plasma concentration of cimetidine (Tagamet) is 1.0 μg/mL; at 2.3 h the concentration is 0.5 μg/mL. Therefore, the concentration of cimetidine decreased to one-half its initial value in 2.3 h—its half-life value. The half-life is independent of the drug concentration and dose administered. In addition, elimination usually occurs according to first-order kinetics: a linear relationship is obtained when the drug concentration is plotted on a *logarithmic* scale versus time on an *arithmetic* scale (a semilogarithmic plot).

11. The answer is C. *(DiPalma, 3/e. p 46.)* The fractional change in drug concentration per unit time is expressed by the elimination rate constant, k_e. This constant is related to half-life ($t_{1/2}$) by the equation

$$k_e t_{1/2} = 0.693$$

The units of the elimination rate constant are time^{-1}, while the $t_{1/2}$ is expressed in units of time. By substitution of the appropriate value for half-life derived from the graph (beta phase) into the above equation, rearranged to solve for k_e, the answer is calculated as follows:

$$k_e = \frac{0.693}{t_{1/2}} = \frac{0.693}{2.3\ \text{h}} = 0.3\ \text{h}^{-1}$$

12. The answer is D. *(DiPalma, 3/e. pp 47–48.)* In the example given, a hypothetical plasma concentration of the drug at zero time (1.8 μg/mL) can be estimated by extrapolating the linear portion of the elimination curve (beta phase) back to zero time. The apparent volume of distribution is the volume of fluid into which the drug appears to distribute or the volume necessary to dissolve the drug and yield the same concentration as that found in plasma. The apparent volume of distribution (V_d) is calculated by

$$V_d = \frac{\text{Total amount of drug in the body}}{\text{Drug concentration in plasma at zero time}}$$

$$V_d = \frac{300\ \text{mg}}{1.8\ \mu\text{g/mL}} = 111\ \text{L}$$

13. The answer is A. *(DiPalma, 3/e. pp 48–49.)* The total body clearance (CL_{total}) is the product of the volume distribution of the drug (V_d) and the elimination rate constant (k_e). It is an expression of the volume of the V_d cleared per unit time. The more rapidly a drug is cleared, the greater is the value of CL_{total}.

$$CL_{total} = V_d k_e = (111\ L)(0.3\ h^{-1}) = 33.5\ L/h$$

14. The answer is D. *(DiPalma, 3/e. pp 52–59. Gilman, 8/e. pp 13–17.)* Biotransformation reactions involving the oxidation, reduction, or hydrolysis of a drug are classified as phase I (or nonsynthetic) reactions; these chemical reactions may result in either the activation or inactivation of a pharmacologic agent. There are many types of these reactions; oxidations are the most numerous. Phase II (or synthetic) reactions, which almost always result in the formation of an inactive product, involve conjugation of the drug (or its derivative) with an amino acid, carbohydrate, acetate, or sulfate. The conjugated form(s) of the drug or its derivatives may be more easily excreted than the parent compound.

15. The answer is D. *(DiPalma, 3/e. pp 37, 49–50, 64. Katzung, 4/e. pp 32–33.)* Bioavailability is defined as the fraction or percentage of a drug that becomes available to the systemic circulation following administration by any route. This takes into consideration that not all of an orally administered drug is absorbed and that a drug can be removed from the plasma and biotransformed by the liver during its initial passage through the portal circulation. A bioavailability of 25 percent indicates that only 20 mg of the 80 mg dose (i.e., 80 mg × 0.25 = 20 mg) reached the systemic circulation. Organ clearance can be determined by knowing the blood flow through the organ (Q) and the extraction ratio (ER) for the drug by the organ, according to the equation

$$CL_{organ} = (Q) \times (ER)$$

The extraction ratio is dependent upon the amounts of drug entering (C_i) and exiting (C_o) the organ; i.e.,

$$ER = \frac{(C_i) - (C_o)}{(C_i)}$$

In this problem the amount of verapamil entering the liver was 76 mg (80 mg × 0.95) and the amount leaving was 20 mg. Therefore,

$$ER = \frac{76\ mg - 20\ mg}{76\ mg} = 0.74$$

$$CL_{liver} = (1500\ mL/min)(0.74) = 1110\ mL/min$$

16. The answer is A. *(AMA Drug Evaluations Annual 1991, 7/e. pp 4, 10–11, 14–15.)* When a new chemical entity is first synthesized by a pharmaceutical company, it is given a *chemical name,* e.g., acetylsalicylic acid. During the process of investigation of the usefulness of the new chemical as a drug, it is given a *generic name* by the United States Adopted Names (USAN) Council, which negotiates with the pharmaceutical manufacturer in the choice of a meaningful and distinctive generic name for the new drug. This name will be the established, official name that can only be applied to that one unique drug compound, e.g., aspirin. The *trade name* (or *brand name,* or *proprietary name*) is a registered name given to the product by the pharmaceutical company that is manufacturing or distributing the drug and identifies a particular product containing that drug, e.g., Ecotrin. Thus, *acetylsalicylic acid, aspirin,* and *Ecotrin,* for example, all refer to the same therapeutic drug entity; however, only *aspirin* is the official generic name.

17. The answer is E. *(DiPalma, 3/e. p 36.)* Tasteless enteric-coated tablets and capsules are formulated to resist the acidic pH found in the stomach. Once the preparation has passed into the intestine, the coating dissolves in the alkaline milieu and releases the drug. Therefore, gastric irritation, drug destruction by gastric acid, and the forming of complexes of the drug with food constituents will be avoided.

18. The answer is C. *(DiPalma, 3/e. pp 16–29.)* There are four major classes of receptors: (1) ion channel receptors, (2) receptors coupled to G-proteins, (3) receptors with tyrosine-specific kinase activity, and (4) receptors for steroid hormones. In most cases, drugs that act via receptors do so by binding to extracellular receptors that transduce the information intracellularly by a variety of mechanisms. Activated ion channel receptors enhance the influx of extracellular ions into the cell; for example, the nicotinic-II cholinergic receptor selectively opens a channel for sodium ions and the $GABA_A$ receptor functions as an ionophore for chloride ions. Receptors coupled to G-proteins (i.e., guanine nucleotide binding proteins) act either by opening an ion channel or by stimulating or inhibiting specific enzymes (e.g., β-adrenergic receptor stimulation leads to an increase in cellular adenylate cyclase activity). When stimulated, receptors with tyrosine-specific protein kinase activity activate this enzyme to enhance the transport of ions and nutrients across the cell membrane; for example, insulin receptors function in this manner and increase glucose transport into insulin-dependent tissues. Steroid hormone receptors are different from all the above in that they are associated with the nucleus of the cell and are activated by steroid hormones (e.g., hydrocortisone) that penetrate into target cells. These receptors interact with DNA to enhance genetic transcription.

19. The answer is E. *(DiPalma, 3/e. pp 40–41. Gilman, 8/e. pp 11–12.)* Since only the free (unbound) fraction of drug can cross biologic membranes, binding to plasma proteins limits a drug's concentration in tissues and therefore decreases the apparent volume of distribution of the drug. Plasma protein binding will also reduce glomerular filtration of the drug since this process is highly dependent on the free drug fraction. Renal tubular secretion and biotransformation of drugs are generally not limited by plasma protein binding because these processes reduce the free drug concentration in the plasma. If a drug is avidly transported through the tubule by the secretion process or rapidly biotransformed, the rates of these processes may exceed the rate of dissociation of the drug-protein complex (in order to restore the free:bound drug ratio in plasma) and thus becomes the rate-limiting factor for drug elimination. This assumes that equilibrium conditions exist and other influences, e.g., changes in pH or the presence of other drugs, do not occur.

20. The answer is C. *(Gilman, 8/e. pp 13, 352–354, 425–426, 650, 661, 760, 801.)* Prodrugs are pharmacologically inactive compounds that, after administration, are converted to an active drug. All the drugs listed are biotransformed to active products; however, only diazepam itself is active and, therefore, is not a prodrug. Diazepam, an active anxiolytic, can be converted to at least three active products: desmethyldiazepam (nordazepam), 3-hydroxydiazepam, and oxazepam (Serax), the last marketed as an antianxiety drug. Minoxidil is oxidized to minoxidil N-O sulfate, the active vasodilator antihypertensive; enalapril is hydrolyzed to form enalaprilat, a potent angiotensin converting enzyme inhibitor; sulfasalazine is cleaved to release its active component mesalamine, an anti-inflammatory agent used for its local action on the bowel; and sulindac is reduced to sulindac sulfide, a nonsteroidal anti-inflammatory drug.

21. The answer is D. *(DiPalma, 3/e. pp 12–13. Gilman, 8/e. pp 45–46.)* Competitive antagonists produce a parallel shift in the dose-response curve of an agonist with no reduction in maximal effect; this is exemplified in the curve shown for norepinephrine plus drug X. Noncompetitive antagonism, as shown with norepinephrine plus drug Y, results in a nonparallel shift in the agonistic dose-response curve and a diminution of the maximum response. Whether X is more potent or more effective than Y as an antagonist cannot be measured by these data.

22. The answer is E. *(Gilman, 8/e. pp 4–5. Katzung, 4/e. pp 2–3.)* Weak acids and weak bases are dissociated into nonionized and ionized forms depending upon the pK_a of the molecule and the pH of the environment. The nonionized form of a drug passes through cellular membranes more easily than the ionized form because it is more lipid-soluble. Thus, the rate of passive transport varies with the proportion of the drug that is nonionized. When the pH of the environment in which a weak acid or weak base drug is contained is equal to the pK_a, the drug is 50 percent dissociated. Weak acids (e.g., salicylates, barbiturates) are more readily absorbed from the stomach than from other regions of the alimentary canal because a large percentage of these weak acids are in the nonionized state. The magnitude of this effect can be estimated by applying the Henderson-Hasselbalch equation:

$$\log\left(\frac{\text{Protonated form}}{\text{Unprotonated form}}\right) = pK_a - pH$$

At an acidic pH of about 3, of the drugs in question all are weak acids except propranolol; therefore, propanolol has the greatest percentage of its molecules in the ionized form in the stomach. The higher the value of the pK_a, the less ionized these substances are in the stomach.

23–25. The answers are: 23-C, 24-D, 25-A. *(Gilman, 8/e. pp 229, 358, 1054, 1119. Katzung, 4/e. pp 12–13, 16–17.)* A therapeutic drug interaction that reduces drug effectiveness results when two drugs with opposing pharmacologic effects are administered. For example, isoproterenol, a β-adrenergic stimulator, will antagonize the effect of propranolol, a β-adrenergic blocking agent. The combined use of amobarbital and secobarbital, both barbiturate sedative-hypnotics, represents a drug interaction that causes an *additive* (enhanced) pharmacologic response, i.e., depression of the central nervous system. The combination of the antimicrobials sulfamethoxazole and trimethoprim (Bactrim, Septra) is an example of a very useful drug interaction in which one drug *potentiates* the effects of another.

Physical interactions result when precipitation or another change in the physical state or solubility of a drug occurs. A common physical drug interaction takes place in the mixture of oppositely charged organic molecules, e.g., cationic (benzalkonium chloride) and anionic (soap) detergents.

Chemical drug interactions result when two administered substances combine with each other chemically. Tetracyclines complex with calcium (in milk), with aluminum and magnesium (often components of antacids), and with iron (in some multiple vitamins) to reduce the absorption of the tetracycline antibiotic.

26–28. The answers are: 26-E, 27-B, 28-A. *(DiPalma, 3/e, pp 12, 335. Katzung, 4/e. pp 25, 727–728.)* Anaphylaxis refers to an acute hypersensitivity reaction that appears to be mediated primarily by IgE. Specific antigens can interact with these antibodies and cause sensitized mast cells to release vasoactive substances, such as histamine. Anaphylaxis to penicillin is one of the best known examples; the drug of choice to relieve the symptoms is epinephrine.

Decreased sensitivity to a drug, or tolerance, is seen with some drugs such as opiates and usually requires repeated administration of the drug. Tachyphylaxis, in contrast, is tolerance that develops rapidly, often after a single injection of drug. In some cases this may be due to what is termed the *down regulation* of drug receptors, in which the number of receptors becomes decreased.

A person who responds to an unusually low dose of a drug is called *hyperreactive*. Supersensitivity refers to increased responses to low doses only after denervation of an organ. At least three mechanisms are responsible for supersensitivity: increased receptors, reduction in tonic neuronal activity, and decreased neurotransmitter uptake mechanisms.

29–33. The answers are: 29-H, 30-C, 31-G, 32-E, 33-A. *(DiPalma, 3/e. pp 96, 121, 224, 255, 267, 301, 309, 539.)* The steroid nucleus, exemplified by prednisone, is shown in Figure A. This is the structural basis for androgens, estrogens, progestogens, and anti-inflammatory corticosteroids.

Figure B is aspirin, a compound that can be categorized as a nonsteroidal anti-inflammatory drug, a nonopioid analgesic, and an antipyretic. Chemically, aspirin belongs to a group of compounds known as salicylates, which includes drugs such as salicylic acid, methylsalicylate, and salsalate.

Figure C illustrates codeine, a derivative of morphine, which contains the pentacyclic opioid structure. Although principally important for their analgesic activity, many opioids are also useful as antidiarrheals, respiratory depressants, and cough suppressants.

Amitriptyline is shown in Figure D. This compound is a member of a large group of compounds known as *tricyclic antidepressants*. The three-ring structure is similar to that of the phenothiazines (Figure G), but the pharmacologic properties are quite different. Other drugs included in this group are imipramine, desipramine, trimipramine, doxepin, and nortriptyline.

Figure E is the compound cephalexin, an important antimicrobial in the treatment of systemic bacterial infections. The four-membered β-lactam ring found in all the cephalosporin antibiotics is also contained within the structure of the penicillin derivatives.

Figure F represents a group of compounds known as *lysergic acid derivatives*, or *ergot alkaloids*, since all are derived from ergot, which is a product of a fungal infestation of grains, particularly rye. The compound shown is ergotamine, a useful vasoconstrictor and a drug used for relieving migraine headaches. Other ergot derivatives include ergonovine (an oxytocic) and bromocriptine (a drug used in the treatment of Parkinson's disease and hyperprolactinemia). These compounds are also structurally related to lysergic acid diethylamide (LSD).

Figure G is the phenothiazine nucleus, attachments to the nitrogen atom of which account principally for the differences in the pharmacokinetics of the various compounds that comprise this group. Examples include the piperazines, such as trifluoperazine; the piperidines, such as thioridazine; and the propylamines, or open-chain compounds, such as chlorpromazine. All of these agents are effective antipsychotic drugs.

Figure H is isoproterenol, a representative of a large class of sympathomimetic compounds, many of which are catecholamine derivatives that stimulate β-adrenergic receptors in bronchiolar smooth muscle, thus inducing the bronchioles to relax. Isoproterenol and structurally similar compounds (epinephrine, albuterol, terbutaline, metaproterenol, and isoetharine) are important bronchodilators used in the therapy of chronic obstructive pulmonary diseases, such as bronchial asthma.

Lorazepam is shown in Figure I. This antianxiety drug is representative of the benzodiazepines, compounds with antianxiety, anticonvulsant, skeletal muscle relaxant, and sedative properties.

Although it is not necessary to know the exact structure of each drug, knowledge of the basic structural characteristics of each class of drugs helps to categorize information and to predict the general properties and effects of some new compounds as they occur.

34–36. The answers are: 34-C, 35-A, 36-H. *(DiPalma, 3/e. pp 6–7.)* Time-action curves relate the changes in intensity of the action of a drug dose and the times that these changes occur. There are three distinct phases that characterize the time-action pattern of most drugs: (1) The *time to onset of action* is from the moment of administration (T on the figure) to the time when the first drug effect is detected (U). (2) The *time to reach the peak effect* is from administration (T) until the maximum effect has occurred (W), regardless of whether this is above or below the level that produces some toxic effect. (3) The *duration of action* is described as the time from the appearance of a drug effect (U) until the effect disappears (Y). For some drugs a fourth phase occurs (interval Y to Z), in which *residual effects* of the drug may be present. These are usually undetectable, but may be uncovered by readministration of the same drug dose (observed as an increase in potency) or by administration of another drug (leading to some drug-drug interaction).

37–39. The answers are: 37-B, 38-A, 39-E. *(DiPalma, 3/e. pp 33–35.)* The absorption, distribution, and elimination of drugs require that they cross various cellular membranes. The descriptions given in the question define the various transport mechanisms. The most common method by which ionic compounds of low molecular weight (100 to 200) enter cells is via membrane channels. The degree to which such filtration occurs varies from cell type to cell type because their pore sizes differ.

Simple diffusion is another mechanism by which substances cross membranes without the active participation of components in the membranes.

Generally, lipid-soluble substances employ this method to enter cells. Both simple diffusion and filtration are dominant factors in most drug absorption, distribution, and elimination.

Carrier-mediated transport provides selectivity to the uptake process and is used to describe both active transport and facilitated diffusion. Active transport is responsible for the movement of a number of organic acids and bases across membranes of renal tubules, choroid plexuses, and hepatic cells. In contrast to active transport, facilitated diffusion does not require energy and so cannot prevail against a concentration gradient. Glucose transport into erythrocytes is a good example of this.

Pinocytosis is a type of endocytosis that is responsible for the transport of large molecules such as proteins and colloids. Some cell types—for example, endothelial cells—employ this transport mechanism extensively, but its importance in drug action is uncertain.

40–42. The answers are: 40-G, 41-A, 42-D. *(DiPalma, 3/e. pp 53–57. Katzung, 4/e. p 43.)* There are four major components to the mixed-function oxidase system: (1) cytochrome P-450, (2) NADPH, or reduced nicotinamide adenine dinucleotide phosphate, (3) NADPH–cytochrome P-450 reductase, and (4) molecular oxygen. The figure shows the catalytic cycle for the reactions dependent upon cytochrome P-450.

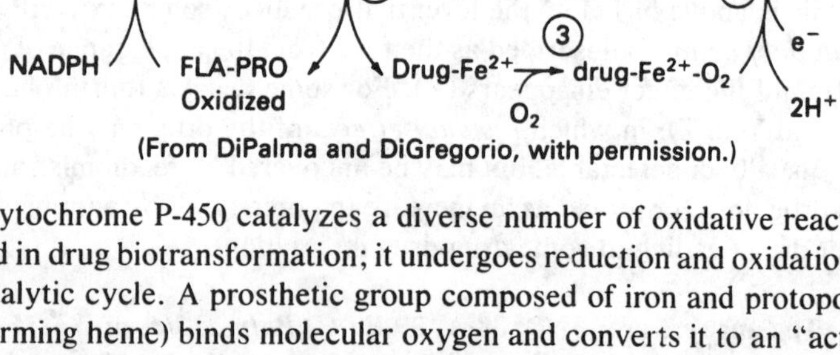

(From DiPalma and DiGregorio, with permission.)

Cytochrome P-450 catalyzes a diverse number of oxidative reactions involved in drug biotransformation; it undergoes reduction and oxidation during its catalytic cycle. A prosthetic group composed of iron and protoporphyrin IX (forming heme) binds molecular oxygen and converts it to an "activated" form for interaction with the drug substrate. Similar to hemoglobin, cytochrome P-450 is inhibited by carbon monoxide. This interaction results in an absorbance spectrum peak at 450 nm, hence the name *P-450*.

NADPH gives up hydrogen atoms to the flavoprotein NADPH–cytochrome P-450 reductase and becomes $NADP^+$. The reduced flavoprotein transfers these reducing equivalents to cytochrome P-450. The reducing equivalents are used to activate molecular oxygen for incorporation into the substrate, as described above. Thus NADPH provides the reducing equivalents, while NADPH–cytochrome P-450 reductase passes them on to the catalytic enzyme cytochrome P-450.

Monoamine oxidase is a flavoprotein enzyme that is found on the outer membrane of mitochondria. It oxidatively deaminates short-chain monoamines only and it is not part of the DMMS. Adenosine triphosphate (ATP) is involved in transfer of reducing equivalents through the mitochondrial respiratory chain, not the microsomal system.

Anti-Infectives

Note: In the classification of drugs in this and subsequent chapters, prototype drugs are marked with an asterisk.

- General Concepts: β-Lactam Antibiotics
  - Cell-wall synthesis
    - Inhibition by β-lactam antibiotics
  - Autolytic enzyme activity
    - Autolysin-deficient bacteria
  - Penicillin-binding proteins (PBPs)
  - Mechanisms of resistance
    - Permeability barrier
    - β-Lactamase production
- Penicillins
  - Natural penicillins
    - Penicillin G*
    - Penicillin V
  - Penicillinase-resistant
    - Methacillin
    - Nafcillin
    - Oxacillin
    - Cloxacillin
    - Dicloxacillin
  - Aminopenicillins
    - Ampicillin*
    - Amoxicillin
  - Extended-spectrum
    - Carbenicillin
    - Ticarcillin
    - Azlocillin
    - Mezlocillin
    - Piperacillin
- β-Lactamase Inhibitors
  - Clavulanic acid*
  - Sulbactam
- Cephalosporins
  - First generation
    - Parenteral use
      - Cefazolin
      - Cephalothin*
      - Cephapirin
      - Cephradine
    - Oral use
      - Cephalexin*
      - Cefadroxil
      - Cephradine
  - Second generation
    - Parenteral use
      - Cefuroxime*
      - Cefamandole
      - Cefonicid
      - Ceforanide
      - Cefoxitin
      - Cefotetan
    - Oral use
      - Cefaclor*
      - Cefuroxime
  - Third generation
    - Parenteral use
      - Cefotaxime*
      - Ceftizoxime
      - Cefoperazone
      - Ceftriaxone
      - Moxalactam
    - Oral use
      - Cefixime
      - Carbapenems
      - Imipenem-cilastatin
    - Monobactams
      - Aztreonam
- Miscellaneous Antibiotics
  - Primarily against gram-positives
    - Erythromycin
    - Vancomycin*
  - Primarily against anaerobes
    - Clindamycin*
    - Metronidazole*
  - Primarily against gram-negatives
    - Streptomycin*

Gentamicin
Tobramycin
Amikacin
Ciprofloxacin
Norfloxacin
Primarily for *N. gonorrhoeae*
Spectinomycin (not an aminoglycoside)
Broad-Spectrum Antimicrobials
Chloramphenicol*
Tetracyclines*
Tetracycline
Oxytetracycline
Demeclocycline
Methacycline
Doxycycline
Minocycline
Sulfonamides
Sulfisoxazole
Sulfadiazine*
Sulfamethoxazole
Sulfamerazine
Sulfamethazine
Sulfamethizole
Sulfameter
Trimethoprim*
Trimethoprim-sulfamethoxazole*
Antituberculosis drugs
Isoniazid*
Rifampin*
Ethambutol*
Pyrazinamide
Streptomycin*
Ethionamide
Capreomycin
Kanamycin
Para-aminosalicylic acid (PAS)
Drugs for leprosy
Dapsone*
Clofazimine
Antimycotic drugs
Amphotericin B*
Nystatin*
Flucytosine*
Griseofulvin*
Ketoconazole*
Miconazole
Antiviral drugs
Amantadine*
Acyclovir*
Vidarabine
Trifluridine
Idoxuridine*
Ribavirin
Zidovudine*
Protozoan infections
Malaria
Quinine, mefloquine*
Chloroquine*
Primaquine*
Proguanil
Pyrimethamine*
Trimethoprim
Sulfonamides
Qinghaosu, artemisinine
Amebiasis
Diloxanide furoate*
Metronidazole*
Tinidazole
Emetine*
Dehydroemetine
Iodoquinol*
Paromomycin
Carbarsone
Chloroquine
Leishmaniasis
Sodium stibogluconate*
Amphotericin B*
Metronidazole*
Allopurinol
Nifurtimox
Trypanosomiasis
Pentamidine
Melarsoprol
Nifurtimox
Suramin
Giardiasis
Metronidazole
Quinacrine
Furazolidone
Trichomoniasis
Metronidazole
Toxoplasmosis
Pyrimethamine-sulfadiazine

Pneumonia caused by *P. carinii*
- Trimethoprim-sulfamethoxazole
- Pentamidine

Antihelmintics
- Mebendazole
- Diethylcarbamazine
- Pyrantel
- Thiabendazole
- Piperazine
- Quinacrine
- Niclosamide
- Oxamniquine
- Praziquantel

DIRECTIONS: Each question below contains five suggested responses. Select the **one best** response to each question.

43. Kernicterus in newborn or premature infants treated with sulfonamides is due to

(A) enhanced synthesis of bilirubin
(B) displacement of bound bilirubin from albumin
(C) inhibition of bilirubin degradation
(D) inhibition of urinary excretion of bilirubin
(E) deposition of crystalline aggregates in the kidneys

44. Aluminum and calcium salts inhibit the intestinal absorption of which of the following agents?

(A) Isoniazid
(B) Chloramphenicol
(C) Phenoxymethyl penicillin
(D) Erythromycin
(E) Tetracycline

45. The drug most effective against malarial parasites in the liver but not effective against parasites within erythrocytes is

(A) primaquine
(B) pyrimethamine
(C) quinacrine
(D) chloroquine
(E) chloroguanide

46. Norfloxacin acid, a quinolone derivative, is

(A) effective in the treatment of urinary tract infections
(B) effective in preventing cell-wall synthesis
(C) ineffective against *Pseudomonas aeruginosa*
(D) only administered parenterally
(E) a nonhalogenated derivative

47. Sulfonamides specifically inhibit which of the following processes?

(A) Conversion of tetrahydrofolic acid to dihydrofolic acid
(B) Conversion of folic acid to folinic acid
(C) Synthesis of DNA
(D) Synthesis of folic acid
(E) Reduction of ribonucleotides

48. The elimination half-life of which of the following tetracyclines remains unchanged when the drug is administered to an anuric patient?

(A) Methacycline
(B) Oxytetracycline
(C) Doxycycline
(D) Tetracycline
(E) None of the above

49. In the treatment of gonococcal infection resistant to penicillins in adults, the drug of choice is

(A) aqueous crystalline penicillin G
(B) benzathine penicillin G
(C) penicillin VK
(D) erythromycin
(E) ceftriaxone

50. In patients with hepatic coma, decreases in the production and absorption of ammonia from the gastrointestinal tract will be beneficial. The antibiotic of choice in this situation would be

(A) neomycin
(B) tetracycline
(C) penicillin G
(D) chloramphenicol
(E) cephalothin

51. Indicate from the diagram below the site of action of penicillinase.

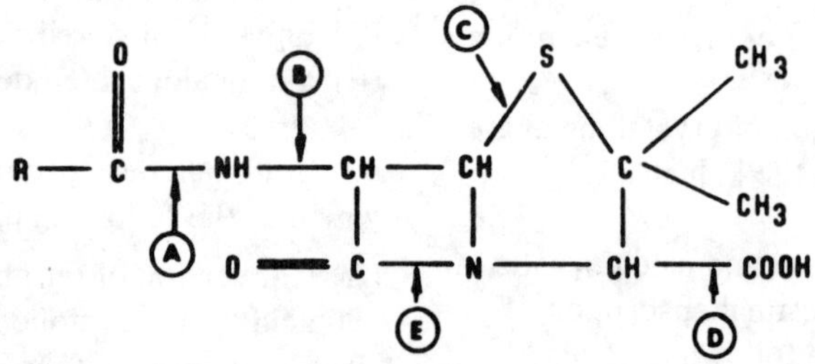

(A) A
(B) B
(C) C
(D) D
(E) E

52. Clavulanic acid is important because it

(A) easily penetrates gram-negative microorganisms
(B) is specific for gram-positive microorganisms
(C) is a potent inhibitor of cell wall transpeptidase
(D) inactivates bacterial β-lactamases
(E) has a spectrum of activity similar to that of penicillin G

53. In the treatment of infections caused by *Pseudomonas aeruginosa,* the antimicrobial agent that has proved to be effective is

(A) penicillin G
(B) piperacillin
(C) nafcillin
(D) erythromycin
(E) tetracycline

54. All the following statements regarding the extended-spectrum penicillins are true EXCEPT

(A) mezlocillin and piperacillin are drugs in this category
(B) they are effective against gram-negative bacilli
(C) they are susceptible to staphylococcal penicillinase
(D) they are the drug of choice for "strep" throat
(E) they produce cross-sensitization with the natural penicillins

55. Ethambutol is administered concurrently with other antitubercular drugs in the treatment of tuberculosis in order to

(A) reduce the pain of injection
(B) facilitate penetration of the blood-brain barrier
(C) retard the development of organism resistance
(D) delay excretion of other antitubercular drugs by the kidney
(E) retard absorption after intramuscular injection

56. The aminoglycoside most likely to remain a useful therapeutic agent in the event of resistance to gentamicin is

(A) streptomycin
(B) amikacin
(C) neomycin
(D) tobramycin
(E) kanamycin

57. The drug used in all types of tuberculosis is

(A) ethambutol
(B) cycloserine
(C) streptomycin
(D) isoniazid
(E) *p*-aminosalicylic acid

58. Candidiasis of the vagina, gastrointestinal tract, and oral cavity is treated primarily by

(A) nystatin
(B) miconazole
(C) rifampin
(D) griseofulvin
(E) iodide

59. Isoniazid, one of the most active drugs for the treatment of tuberculosis,

(A) cannot be used with rifampin or ethambutol
(B) works primarily by preventing protein synthesis
(C) possesses toxicities that can be prevented by pyridoxine
(D) is removed from the body unchanged
(E) is rarely met with resistance to its action

60. For the treatment of a patient with *Legionella* pneumonia, the drug of choice would be

(A) penicillin G
(B) chloramphenicol
(C) erythromycin
(D) streptomycin
(E) lincomycin

61. The most effective agent in the treatment of *Rickettsia, Mycoplasma,* and *Chlamydia* infections is

(A) penicillin G
(B) tetracycline
(C) vancomycin
(D) gentamicin
(E) bacitracin

62. All the following antibiotics inhibit bacterial cell wall synthesis EXCEPT

(A) bacitracin
(B) cycloserine
(C) cephalothin
(D) vancomycin
(E) polymyxins

63. The mechanism of action by which niclosamide is effective against adult intestinal cestodes is

(A) interference with cell-wall synthesis
(B) interference with cell division
(C) inhibition of mitochondrial oxidative phosphorylation
(D) interference with protein synthesis
(E) depletion of membrane lipoproteins

64. All the following penicillins are resistant to penicillinase EXCEPT

(A) oxacillin
(B) cloxacillin
(C) ticarcillin
(D) nafcillin
(E) dicloxacillin

65. Vertigo, inability to perceive termination of movement, and difficulty in sitting or standing without visual clues are some of the toxic reactions that are likely to occur in about 75 percent of patients who

(A) are allergic to penicillin
(B) receive tetracycline therapy
(C) receive amphotericin B therapy
(D) receive streptomycin therapy
(E) receive isoniazid therapy for tuberculosis

66. Amantadine (Symmetrel), a synthetic antiviral agent used prophylactically against influenza A_2, is thought to act by

(A) preventing production of viral capsid protein
(B) preventing virion release
(C) preventing penetration of the virus into the host cell
(D) preventing synthesis of nucleic acid
(E) causing lysis of infected host cells by release of intracellular lysosomal enzymes

67. Streptomycin and other aminoglycosides inhibit bacterial protein synthesis by binding

(A) peptidoglycan units in the cell wall
(B) messenger RNA
(C) DNA
(D) 30S ribosomal particles
(E) RNA polymerase

68. Which of the following statements concerning griseofulvin is true?

(A) It inhibits the growth of dermatophytes
(B) It inhibits synthesis of the cell wall
(C) It inhibits synthesis of the cell membrane
(D) It is used primarily as a short-term drug
(E) It is administered primarily by the parenteral route

69. Quinine, an antimalarial drug, causes all the following EXCEPT

(A) local anesthesia
(B) local destruction of tissue
(C) analgesia
(D) antipyretic effects
(E) hypertension

70. Idoxuridine is a synthetic antiviral agent with all the following properties EXCEPT

(A) a structure containing a halogen atom
(B) activity against DNA viruses
(C) major use in the treatment of herpes simplex keratitis
(D) topical use on the eye
(E) major use in treatment of herpes simplex virus type 2

71. All the following are associated with the use of penicillin EXCEPT

(A) hypersensitization
(B) interstitial nephritis
(C) impaired platelet function
(D) seizures
(E) disulfiram-like reaction

72. Which of the following is a correct statement concerning the pharmacology of spectinomycin?

(A) It interacts with bacterial 50S subunits
(B) It is classified as an aminoglycoside
(C) It is active against *Neisseria gonorrhoeae*
(D) It possesses ototoxicity
(E) It possesses nephrotoxicity

73. All the following statements are true concerning cephalosporins in comparison with penicillins EXCEPT

(A) their structures are closely related
(B) their mechanisms of action are analogous
(C) cephalosporins have an unusually broader antimicrobial spectrum
(D) their hypersensitivity reactions are distinguished by distinct signs and symptoms
(E) cephalosporins can cause bleeding problems related to hypoprothrombinemia

74. Penicillin has little or no antibacterial action against

(A) *Treponema pallidum*
(B) gonococci
(C) meningococci
(D) resting bacterial cells
(E) actively growing bacterial cells

75. Which of the following cephalosporins would have increased activity against anaerobic bacteria such as *Bacteroides fragilis?*

(A) Cefaclor
(B) Cephalothin
(C) Cephalexin
(D) Cefamandole
(E) Cefoxitin

76. Which one of the following antimicrobial agents is primarily administered topically?

(A) Polymyxin B
(B) Penicillin G
(C) Dicloxacillin
(D) Carbenicillin
(E) Streptomycin

77. Streptomycin is an effective aminoglycoside that

(A) is administered orally
(B) is not significantly metabolized
(C) does not accumulate in patients with renal impairment
(D) is used widely against gram-positive enteric bacteria
(E) is ineffective against tuberculosis

78. Which one of the following statements is correct about Vancomycin?

(A) It inhibits cell-wall synthesis
(B) It is primarily effective against gram-negative organisms
(C) It is administered primarily by the oral route
(D) It is the cause of Franconi syndrome
(E) It is the cause of "gray baby syndrome"

79. All the following reactions are associated with the antibiotic moxalactam EXCEPT

(A) hypersensitivity
(B) neutropenia
(C) hypoprothrombinemia
(D) thrombocytopenia
(E) crystalluria

80. Metronidazole is effective in the treatment of all the following EXCEPT

(A) trichomoniasis in females
(B) asymptomatic trichomoniasis in males
(C) giardiasis
(D) infection with *Bacteroides fragilis*
(E) streptococcal infection

81. Common complications of cephalothin therapy in hospitalized patients include all the following EXCEPT

(A) fever, eosinophilia, and anaphylaxis
(B) superinfection with gram-negative organisms
(C) thrombophlebitis
(D) nephrotoxicity
(E) hemolytic anemia

82. Which one of the following penicillins is resistant to penicillinase?

(A) Ampicillin
(B) Oxacillin
(C) Carbenicillin
(D) Ticarcillin
(E) Mezlocillin

83. Correct statements about the clinical application of carbenicillin include which of the following?

(A) It has little activity against gram-negative bacteria
(B) It is ineffective against *Pseudomonas*
(C) It can cause hypokalemic alkalosis
(D) It frequently causes diarrhea
(E) It is resistant to β-lactamase

84. One of the mechanisms associated with bacteria's resistance to penicillin is

(A) ability of bacteria to produce an acid media
(B) bacterial production of lysozymes
(C) alteration of penicillin-binding proteins (PBPs)
(D) increased metabolism of the penicillin
(E) increased renal excretion of penicillins

85. Ketoconazole is a broadly useful antifungal compound that

(A) is usually administered parenterally
(B) possesses androgenic activity
(C) is excellent for infections of the central nervous system
(D) is effective in chronic suppressive therapy for mucocutaneous candidiasis
(E) can cause steroid abnormalities in patients

86. All the following are properties of amphotericin B EXCEPT

(A) it can cause renal and liver dysfunctions
(B) it is poorly absorbed via the oral route
(C) it is used for the treatment of systemic fungal infections
(D) it binds to ergosterol to disturb the fungal membrane
(E) it is a potent inhibitor of cell-wall synthesis

87. Thiabendazole (Mintezol), a benzimidazole derivative, is an anthelmintic drug used primarily to treat infections caused by

(A) *Ascaris*
(B) *Necator americanus* (hookworm)
(C) *Strongyloides*
(D) *Enterobius vermicularis*
(E) *Taenia saginata* (flatworm)

88. Sulfonamides may cause renal damage that has been shown to be the result of precipitation of crystals in the collecting tubules of the kidney. Predisposing factors to such crystal formation include

(A) low urinary concentration of the drug
(B) high urinary solubility of the drug
(C) a urine pH of 5.0
(D) simultaneous administration of several sulfonamides
(E) administration of the drug parenterally

89. The drug of choice in *Plasmodium falciparum* malaria is

(A) quinine
(B) pyrimethamine-sulfadoxine
(C) tetracycline
(D) primaquine
(E) chloroquine

90. All the following statements are true of acyclovir EXCEPT

(A) it is a nucleoside antiviral drug
(B) it converts to a triphosphate and subsequently inhibits synthesis of viral DNA
(C) it is available topically and orally
(D) it is used against herpes simplex
(E) it is an analogue of purine metabolites

91. The use of chloramphenicol may result in

(A) bone marrow stimulation
(B) phototoxicity
(C) aplastic anemia
(D) staining of teeth
(E) alopecia

92. A drug primarily used in pneumonia caused by *Pneumocystis carinii* is

(A) nifurtimox
(B) penicillin G
(C) metronidazole
(D) pentamidine
(E) carbenicillin

93. A third-generation cephalosporin is

(A) cephalexin
(B) cefoperazone
(C) cefoxitin
(D) cephalothin
(E) cefamandole

94. A fresh case of amebic dysentery is most appropriately treated with metronidazole. An accurate characterization of this drug is that it

(A) is the treatment of choice for asymptomatic carriers of cysts
(B) is poorly absorbed from the intestinal tract
(C) has more severe adverse effects than does emetine
(D) is effective in both the intestinal (luminal) and tissue stages of *Entamoeba histolytica*
(E) is ineffective against trichomoniasis

95. One of the reasons aminoglycosides are frequently combined with other antibiotics to treat certain infections is to

(A) prevent drug interactions
(B) prevent the emergence of resistant bacteria
(C) increase renal excretion
(D) increase oral absorption
(E) decrease systemic toxicities

96. Neuromuscular blockade produced by tubocurarine is potentiated by

(A) neomycin
(B) bacitracin
(C) cephalothin
(D) penicillin
(E) chloramphenicol

97. Chloramphenicol, a completely synthetic antibiotic, is the drug of choice in

(A) symptomatic *Salmonella* infections
(B) brucellosis
(C) urinary tract infection by *Escherichia coli*
(D) cholera
(E) streptococcal pharyngitis

98. A true statement concerning cephalosporin antibiotics is which of the following?

(A) Cephalosporins are only bacteriostatic against multiplying bacteria
(B) Cephalosporins and penicillins have dissimilar mechanisms of activity
(C) Cross-hypersensitivity exists between cephalosporins and penicillins
(D) Cephalosporins are resistant to inactivation by β-lactamase
(E) Cephalosporins are usually administered orally

99. A correct statement concerning the reactions caused by aminoglycosides is that these agents

(A) produce ototoxicity
(B) are potent neuromuscular blockers
(C) have little or no effect on kidneys
(D) produce a high incidence of hypersensitivity reactions similar to those of penicillins
(E) produce a high incidence of exfoliated dermatitis

100. A pharmacologic property of amphotericin B is

(A) effective gastrointestinal absorption
(B) usefulness in the treatment of systemic mycoses
(C) binding to DNA
(D) absence of renal toxicity
(E) inhibition of cell-wall synthesis

101. The gray baby syndrome, which is caused by chloramphenicol in the newborn, is

(A) not a serious problem
(B) related to an immature hepatic conjugating mechanism
(C) unrelated to renal function
(D) characterized by life-threatening hyperthermia
(E) associated with hypertension

102. To inhibit the antibacterial activity of sulfonamides, one should administer

(A) acetylsalicylate
(B) folic acid
(C) pantothenic acid
(D) vitamin B_{12}
(E) methotrexate

103. The activity of dihydrofolate reductase is inhibited by

(A) succinylsulfathiazole (Sulfsuxidine)
(B) trimethoprim
(C) sulfamethoxazole (Gantanol)
(D) tetracycline
(E) griseofulvin

DIRECTIONS: Each group of questions below consists of lettered headings followed by a set of numbered items. For each numbered item select the **one** lettered heading with which it is **most** closely associated. Each lettered heading may be used **once, more than once, or not at all.**

Questions 104–107

For each of the antibiotics below, select the appropriate mode of action.

(A) Binds to the 30S ribosome subunit
(B) Inhibits cell-membrane synthesis
(C) Inhibits binding of aminoacyl RNA to the 50S ribosome subunit
(D) Inhibits folic acid reductase
(E) Inhibits production of cell wall
(F) Reversibly binds to the 50S ribosome subunit
(G) Inhibits RNA polymerase
(H) Inhibits synthesis of steroids

104. Streptomycin

105. Erythromycin

106. Penicillin G

107. Chloramphenicol

Questions 108–112

For each of the parasites below, select the drug that is most effective against it.

(A) Bithionol
(B) Methotrexate
(C) Pyrantel pamoate
(D) Penicillin
(E) Praziquantel
(F) Ceftriaxone
(G) Diethylcarbamazine (Hetrazan)
(H) Primaquine
(I) Niclosamide
(J) Chloroquine

108. *Ascaris lumbricoides* (roundworms)

109. Wuchereria bancrofti (filariae)

110. *Fasciola hepatica* (sheep liver flukes)

111. *Taenia saginata* (tapeworms)

112. *Schistosoma haematobium* (blood flukes)

Questions 113–117

For each of the drugs below, select the most suitable description.

(A) Parenteral penicillin that is resistant to β-lactamase
(B) Oral penicillin that is resistant to β-lactamase
(C) Referred to as an extended-spectrum penicillin
(D) Chemically a cephalosporin
(E) Related to ampicillin but with better oral absorption
(F) Administered intramuscularly and yields prolonged drug levels
(G) Cause of a disulfiram-like reaction
(H) Given parenterally and may cause elevation of serum sodium
(I) Cause of hypothrombinemia

113. Benzathine penicillin G

114. Methicillin

115. Piperacillin

116. Amoxicillin

117. Carbenicillin

Anti-Infectives

Answers

43. The answer is B. *(DiPalma, 3/e. p 623. Gilman, 8/e. p 1037.)* Sulfonamides should not be used in neonates, especially premature infants, since the drug competes with bilirubin for serum albumin binding. This results in increased levels of free bilirubin, which cause kernicterus. Pregnant women at term also should not receive sulfonamides because of this drug's ability to cross the placenta and enter the fetus in concentrations sufficient to produce toxic effects.

44. The answer is E. *(DiPalma, 3/e. pp 618–619. Gilman, 8/e. p 1119.)* Tetracyclines, as chelating agents, have a high affinity for the divalent cations of calcium and magnesium salts, for iron-containing preparations, for dairy products, and for aluminum hydroxide gels. The chelated complex is insoluble and not absorbed through the mucosa of the gastrointestinal tract. Tetracyclines should be administered before meals to prevent formation of such chelates. Antacids that contain cations of calcium, magnesium, or aluminum should not be administered simultaneously with tetracyclines. These cations do not affect the absorption of the other drugs listed in the question.

45. The answer is A. *(DiPalma, 3/e. pp 653–654. Gilman, 8/e. pp 988–989.)* Primaquine is very active against exoerythrocytic forms of *Plasmodium vivax* and *P. falciparum*. While it exhibits some activity against asexual blood forms of *P. vivax*, results are variable. It is completely ineffective against asexual blood forms of *P. falciparum*. Primaquine is the agent of choice against late tissue forms of vivax malaria.

46. The answer is A. *(DiPalma, 3/e. pp 613–615. Gilman, 8/e. pp 1059–1060.)* Norfloxacin is a fluorinated quinoline derivative designed specifically for urinary tract infections. It causes interference of DNA gyrase and ultimately replication. Norfloxacin is administered orally for infections produced by various organisms, including *Pseudomonas aeruginosa*.

47. The answer is D. *(DiPalma, 3/e. pp 621–622. Gilman, 8/e. p 1048.)* Sulfonamides, structural analogues of para-aminobenzoic acid, specifically inhibit the synthesis of folic acid. This in turn leads to inhibition of protein, RNA, and DNA synthesis and to concomitant cessation of growth because folic acid in its cofactor form is required for the synthesis of all these macromolecules. The fact that human cells do not contain folic acid synthetase is the basis for the selective toxicity of the sulfonamides.

48. The answer is C. *(DiPalma, 3/e. p 619. Gilman, 8/e. p 1120.)* All tetracyclines can produce negative nitrogen balance and increased blood urea nitrogen (BUN) levels. This is of clinical importance in patients with impaired renal function. With the exception of doxycycline, tetracyclines should not be used in patients that are anuric. Doxycycline is excreted by the gastrointestinal tract under these conditions and it will not accumulate in the serum of patients with renal insufficiency.

49. The answer is E. *(DiPalma, 3/e. pp 598. Gilman, 8/e. p 1073.)* The penicillins are primary agents in the treatment of syphilis and gonorrhea. However, due to the increased prevalence of resistant strains of *Neisseria gonorrhoeae*, ceftriaxone is considered to be the drug of choice for these organisms. The drug can be given in a single dose intramuscularly. Aqueous procaine penicillin G provides the convenience of single-dose therapy, but possible procaine reaction or penicillin anaphylaxis must be considered.

50. The answer is A. *(Gilman, 8/e. p 1112.)* Neomycin, an aminoglycoside, is not significantly absorbed from the gastrointestinal tract. After oral administration, the intestinal flora is suppressed or modified and the drug is excreted in the feces. This effect of neomycin is used in hepatic coma to decrease the coliform flora, thus decreasing the production of ammonia causing the levels of free nitrogen to decrease in the bloodstream. Other antimicrobial agents—such as tetracycline, penicillin G, chloramphenicol, and cephalothin—do not have the potency of neomycin in causing this effect.

51. The answer is E. *(DiPalma, 3/e. pp 583–584. Gilman, 8/e. pp 1066–1067.)* Penicillinase hydrolyzes the β-lactam ring of penicillin G to form inactive penicillonic acid. Consequently, the antibiotic is ineffective in the therapy of infections caused by penicillinase-producing microorganisms such as staphylococci, bacilli, *Escherichia coli*, *Pseudomonas aeruginosa*, and *Mycobacterium tuberculosis*.

52. The answer is D. *(DiPalma, 3/e. pp 591–592. Gilman, 8/e. p 1093.)* The antibiotic clavulanic acid is a potent inhibitor of β-lactamases. The mode of inhibition is irreversible. Although clavulanic acid does not effectively inhibit the transpeptidase, it may be used in conjunction with a β-lactamase-sensitive penicillin to potentiate its activity.

53. The answer is B. *(DiPalma, 3/e. p 590. Gilman, 8/e. p 1069.)* Piperacillin is a broad-spectrum, semisynthetic penicillin for parenteral use. Its spectrum of activity includes various gram-positive and gram-negative organisms including *Pseudomonas*. The indications for piperacillin are similar to those for carbenicillin, ticarcillin, and mezlocillin with the primary use being suspected or proven infections caused by *P. aeruginosa*. Penicillin G, nafcillin, erythromycin, and tetracycline are ineffective against *Pseudomonas*.

54. The answer is D. *(DiPalma, 3/e. pp 590–591. Gilman, 8/e. p 1069.)* The extended-spectrum penicillins, which include mezlocillin, azlocillin, and piperacillin, have a broad spectrum of activity against gram-negative bacilli. All are susceptible to staphylococcal penicillinase and must be administered parenterally since they are not absorbed from the gastrointestinal tract. Major toxicity includes the penicillin hypersensitization reaction. They are used only in severe infections that do not respond to natural penicillins.

55. The answer is C. *(DiPalma, 3/e. p 630. Gilman, 8/e. p 1158.)* An important problem in the chemotherapy of tuberculosis is bacterial drug resistance. For this reason, concurrent administration of two or more drugs should be employed to delay the development of drug resistance. Isoniazid (Nydrazid) is often combined with ethambutol (Myambutol) for this purpose. Streptomycin or rifampin (Rifadin) may also be added to the regimen to delay even further the development of drug resistance.

56. The answer is B. *(DiPalma, 3/e. pp 610–611. Gilman, 8/e. p 1110.)* The most important mechanism of aminoglycoside resistance in bacteria is drug inactivation by microbial enzymes. Amikacin is uniquely resistant to these enzymes and, therefore, has the broadest spectrum of activity of all the aminoglycosides. It is relatively resistant to several enzymes that inactivate gentamicin and tobramycin, and it therefore can be employed against some microorganisms resistant to these drugs.

57. The answer is D. *(DiPalma, 3/e. pp 626–627. Gilman, 8/e. pp 1148–1149.)* Isoniazid is an effective tuberculostatic drug. Only actively growing bacilli are susceptible to the bactericidal property of isoniazid. The major action of isoniazid is on the cell wall of the bacillus, where it prevents the synthesis of mycolic acid.

58. The answer is A. *(DiPalma, 3/e. p 636. Gilman, 8/e. pp 1177–1179.)* Nystatin (Mycostatin) is used primarily to treat candidal infections of the skin, mucous membranes, and intestinal tract. It is too toxic for parenteral use, but a closely related compound, amphotericin B, may be used systemically. Nystatin and amphotericin B interfere with membrane function in sensitive fungi by increasing the membrane's permeability to a number of small molecules. The use of miconazole is restricted to topical application and vaginal fungal infections associated with the tinea organisms. Griseofulvin is used primarily for skin mycoses. Iodide is restricted to topical application.

59. The answer is C. *(DiPalma, 3/e. p 627. Gilman, 8/e. pp 1146–1149.)* Isoniazid is the most widely useful drug in tuberculosis, in combination with rifampin or ethambutol. The mechanism of action of isoniazid involves the inhibition of synthesis of mycolic acids. Isoniazid is metabolized to an acetylated form. Some toxic reactions include peripheral neuritis, insomnia, and restlessness. The peripheral neuritis can be prevented by pretreatment with pyridoxine.

60. The answer is C. *(DiPalma, 3/e. pp 602–603. Gilman, 8/e. pp 1133-1134.)* Erythromycin, a macrolide antibiotic, was initially designed to be used in penicillin-sensitive patients with streptococcal or pneumococcal infections. Erythromycin has become the drug of choice for the treatment of pneumonia caused by *Mycoplasma* and *Legionella*.

61. The answer is B. *(DiPalma, 3/e. pp 617–619. Gilman, 8/e. pp 1123–1124.)* Tetracycline is one of the drugs of choice in the treatment of *Rickettsia, Mycoplasma*, and *Chlamydia* infections. The antibiotics that act by inhibiting cell wall synthesis have no effect on *Mycoplasma* since the organism does not possess a cell wall; penicillin G, vancomycin, and bacitracin will be ineffective. Gentamicin has little or no antimicrobial activity with these organisms.

62. The answer is E. *(DiPalma, 3/e. pp 581–582. Gilman, 8/e. pp 1066, 1139–1140.)* Bacitracin, cycloserine, cephalothin, and vancomycin inhibit cell wall synthesis and produce bacteria susceptible to environmental conditions. Polymyxins disrupt the structural integrity of the cytoplasmic membranes by acting as cationic detergents. On contact with the drug, the permeability of the membrane changes.

63. The answer is C. *(DiPalma, 3/e. pp 672–673. Gilman, 8/e. p 965.)* Niclosamide, an anthelmintic agent, exerts its effect against cestodes via the inhibition of mitochondrial oxidative phosphorylation in the parasites. The mechanism is also related to its inhibition of glucose and oxygen uptake in the parasite. The drug-induced destruction of the parasite's integument may render the cestode susceptible to digestion by the host's intestinal proteolytic enzymes.

64. The answer is C. *(DiPalma, 3/e. pp 590–591. Gilman, 8/e. pp 1075–1077.)* Ticarcillin resembles carbenicillin and has a high degree of potency against *Pseudomonas* and *Proteus* organisms but is broken down by penicillinase produced by various bacteria, including most staphylococci. Oxacillin, cloxacillin, nafcillin, and dicloxacillin are all resistant to penicillinase and are effective against staphylococci.

65. The answer is D. *(DiPalma, 3/e. pp 611–612. Gilman, 8/e. pp 1104–1108.)* Streptomycin and other aminoglycosides can elicit toxic reactions involving both the vestibular and auditory branches of the eighth cranial nerve. Patients receiving an aminoglycoside should be monitored frequently for any hearing impairment owing to the irreversible deafness that may result from its prolonged use. None of the other agents listed in the question adversely affect the function of the eighth cranial nerve.

66. The answer is C. *(DiPalma, 3/e. pp 639–640. Gilman, 8/e. p 1191.)* Amantadine's mechanism of action is not entirely understood, but it appears to block the attachment of the virus to cells. The drug does not affect penetration and RNA-dependent RNA polymerase activity. Amantadine both reduces the frequency of illness and diminishes the serologic response to influenza infection. The drug has no action, however, on influenza B. As a weak base, amantadine buffers the pH of endosomes, thus blocking the fusion of the viral envelope with the membrane of the endosome.

67. The answer is D. *(DiPalma, 3/e. p 609. Gilman, 8/e. p 1100.)* The bactericidal activity of streptomycin and other aminoglycosides involves a direct action on the 30S ribosomal subunit, the site at which these agents both inhibit protein synthesis and diminish the accuracy of translation of the genetic code. Proteins containing improper sequences of amino acids ("nonsense" proteins) are often nonfunctional.

68. The answer is A. *(DiPalma, 3/e. p 637. Gilman, 8/e. pp 1173–1174.)* Griseofulvin is a potent, orally administered antifungal agent effective against various dermatophytes including *Epidermophyton* and *Trichophyton*. The mechanism of action appears to be related to the interference of nucleic acid synthesis and polymerization. When given for a specific fungal infection, griseofulvin must be continued for 3 to 6 weeks if only hair or skin is involved, but 3 to 6 months if nails are affected.

69. The answer is E. *(DiPalma, 3/e. pp 651–652. Gilman, 8/e. pp 991–993.)* Quinine has analgesic and antipyretic properties similar to those of the salicylates. When applied locally, quinine has a local anesthetic action in which it briefly stimulates and then paralyzes sensory neurons. Because of its nature as protoplasmic poison, local destruction of tissue often results, which prolongs its action for weeks or months. When administered intravenously, quinine causes hypotension similar to that of its isomer quinidine.

70. The answer is E. *(DiPalma, 3/e. p 642. Gilman, 8/e. p 1188.)* Idoxuridine is a halogenated derivative of deoxyuridine. Its major action is on the DNA viruses, with little or no effect on RNA viruses. Its major use is in the treatment of herpes simplex keratitis, where it is usually used topically on the eye. When used topically, it may cause local irritation, photophobia, and occlusion of the lacrimal duct. Although effective against herpes simplex keratitis, idoxuridine is unresponsive to other herpes infections, including herpes simplex virus type 2 and varicella-zoster virus.

71. The answer is E. *(DiPalma, 3/e. pp 584–586. Gilman, 8/e. p 1091.)* Allergic reactions are the main adverse effects encountered with the use of the penicillins. Sensitization is usually the result of previous treatment with a penicillin. Penicillins are not nephrotoxic; however, allergic interstitial nephritis may occur, particularly with methicillin. Hematologic reactions caused by penicillins are rare, but high concentrations may impair platelet function, resulting in prolongation of bleeding time. Seizures may develop when high doses of penicillins are given in the presence of renal insufficiency. Intolerance of alcohol (disulfiram-like reaction) has been noted only with certain cephalosporins.

72. The answer is C. *(DiPalma, 3/e. p 613. Katzung, 4/e. pp 575–577.)* Spectinomycin interacts with the bacterial 30S ribosomal subunit to inhibit protein synthesis. It does not cause misreading of polyribonucleotides as do the aminoglycosides. Spectinomycin differs structurally and biologically from the aminoglycosides and does not possess the nephrotoxicity or ototoxicity of the aminoglycosides. Spectinomycin is used to treat acute gonococcal urethritis and proctitis in men when the causative organism is susceptible and the primary drugs are ineffective or cannot be used.

73. The answer is D. *(DiPalma, 3/e. pp 592–598. Gilman, 8/e. pp 1085–1092.)* Cephalosporins and penicillins have similar structures, penicillins having a penicillanic acid and the cephalosporins a cephalosporinic acid moiety. Both groups of antimicrobials inhibit the transpeptidase enzyme necessary for cross-linking. It appears that the mechanism is not totally identical for every drug for every bacterial species. Cephalosporins have a greater overall activity against gram-negative organisms than do the penicillin G–type compounds. The hypersensitivity reactions associated with the penicillins and the cephalosporins appear to be identical in signs and symptoms. There is a crossover sensitivity between the penicillins and cephalosporins that must be considered when a patient is sensitive to either of these antibiotics.

74. The answer is D. *(DiPalma, 3/e. pp 580–582. Katzung, 4/e. pp 545–549.)* Because penicillins have no effect on existing bacterial cell walls, the bacteria must be multiplying in order for the bactericidal action of penicillin to occur. *Treponema pallidum*, gonococci, and meningococci are very susceptible to the action of penicillin G, and in most cases this is the drug of choice for treating infections caused by these organisms.

75. The answer is E. *(DiPalma, 3/e. p 597. Gilman, 8/e. p 1089.)* Cefoxitin and moxalactam are suitable for treating intraabdominal infections. Such infections are caused by mixtures of aerobic and anaerobic gram-negative bacteria like *Bacteroides fragilis*. Cefoxitin alone has been shown to be as effective as the traditional therapy of clindamycin plus gentamicin.

76. The answer is A. *(DiPalma, 3/e. pp 589–590. Gilman, 8/e. pp 1138–1139.)* Polymyxin B is poorly absorbed by the oral route. It is primarily administered by the topical route for the treatment of infections of the skin, mucous membranes, eye, and ear. Penicillin G can be administered both orally and parenterally. Dicloxacillin is only given by the oral route. Carbenicillin and streptomycin are administered only by the parenteral route.

77. The answer is B. *(DiPalma, 3/e. pp 610–613. Gilman, 8/e. pp 1157–1158.)* Streptomycin is poorly absorbed if at all from the gastrointestinal tract. The drug is not broken down in the body and is excreted primarily by the renal route. Therefore, doses must be adjusted in patients with renal disease to prevent accumulation. Streptomycin is very effective against gram-negative enteric bacteria or when there is evidence of sepsis. It is also useful in the treatment of tuberculosis.

78. The answer is A. *(DiPalma, 3/e. p 605. Gilman, 8/e. pp 1138–1140.)* Vancomycin is a bactericidal agent that inhibits cell-wall synthesis. It inhibits the third stage of peptidoglycan synthesis. Virtually all gram-positive bacteria are sensitive to vancomycin; however, the drug has no significant activity against gram-negative organisms. Vancomycin is absorbed poorly from the gastrointestinal tract, so it is administered intravenously. Major toxic reactions include phlebitis, ototoxicity, and nephrotoxicity. Franconi syndrome and "gray baby syndrome" are clinical manifestations of administration of chloramphenicol.

79. The answer is E. *(AMA Drug Evaluations Annual 1991, 7/e. pp 1242–1243. DiPalma, 3/e. pp 594–623.)* Moxalactam along with cefamandole and cefoperazone can suppress the gastrointestinal microflora with resultant decreased vitamin K production and hypoprothrombinemia. Hypersensitivity reactions, neutropenia, nausea, vomiting, and thrombocytopenia are common adverse reactions observed with all the cephalosporins. Crystalluria, particularly in acid urine, occurs primarily with the use of sulfonamide drugs, which can cause renal damage.

80. The answer is E. *(DiPalma, 3/e. pp 607–608. Gilman, 8/e. pp 1002–1003.)* Metronidazole is a low-molecular-weight compound that penetrates all tissues and fluids of the body. Metronidazole's spectrum of activity is limited largely to anaerobic bacteria—including *B. fragilis*—and certain protozoa. It is considered to be the drug of choice for trichomoniasis in females and carrier states in males as well as intestinal infections with *Giardia lamblia*.

81. The answer is E. *(DiPalma, 3/e. pp 594–595. Gilman, 8/e. p 1091.)* In about 5 percent of the patients receiving cephalothin, a hypersensitivity reaction develops that is characterized by fever, eosinophilia, serum sickness, rash, and anaphylaxis. A positive Coombs' test result is also frequent but is seldom associated with hemolytic anemia. Thrombophlebitis with intravenous administration of cephalothin is almost universal. Superinfection by cephalothin-resistant gram-negative bacilli has been noted by several observers. The cephalosporins have also been implicated as potentially nephrotoxic agents.

82. The answer is B. *(DiPalma, 3/e. pp 588–589. Gilman, 8/e. pp 1068–1069.)* Oxacillin is resistant to penicillinase; ampicillin, carbenicillin, ticarcillin, and mezlocillin are not. These latter four agents are broad-spectrum penicillins, while oxacillin is generally specific for gram-positive microorganisms. Use of penicillinase-resistant penicillins should be reserved for infections caused by penicillinase-producing staphylococci.

83. The answer is C. *(DiPalma, 3/e. pp 590–591. Gilman, 8/e. pp 1080–1081.)* Carbenicillin resembles ampicillin but has more activity against *Pseudomonas* and *Proteus* organisms than do the standard penicillin G preparations. Carbenicillin is susceptible to penicillinase (β-lactamase), and its activity is lost when hydrolyzed by this enzyme. One of the unusual effects of carbenicillin is its ability to cause a lowering of total body potassium through a renal mechanism, thus leading to hypokalemic alkalosis. Although some gastrointestinal symptoms have been noted with carbenicillin, ampicillin traditionally has been associated with frequent diarrhea.

84. The answer is C. *(DiPalma, 3/e. pp 582–583. Gilman, 8/e. pp 1067–1068.)* Bacterial resistance to β-lactam (penicillin) antibiotics may be due to one or more of the following mechanisms: inability of the drug to penetrate to the target site of its action; alteration of PBPs resulting in reduced affinity for the drug; and inactivation of the drug by bacterial enzymes known as β-lactamases.

85. The answer is D. *(DiPalma, 3/e. pp 637–638. Gilman, 8/e. p 1171.)* Ketoconazole is readily absorbed from the gastrointestinal tract under acidic conditions. It does not penetrate well into the cerebrospinal fluid, which limits its effectiveness in the treatment of infections of the central nervous system. Ketoconazole has antiandrogenic effects by reducing testosterone synthesis. It is very effective in the treatment of chronic mucocutaneous candidiasis. Ketoconazole inhibits steroid biosynthesis by inhibition of cytochrome P-450.

86. The answer is E. *(DiPalma, 3/e. pp 634–636. Gilman, 8/e. pp 1165–1168.)* Amphotericin B disturbs the permeability and transport mechanisms of membranes by binding to ergosterol in the membrane. It is poorly absorbed via the oral route and must be given parenterally for the treatment of systemic fungal infections. In therapeutic concentrations, amphotericin B has the potential of causing both renal and liver damage, and the dose must be reduced when these toxicities develop. It has little or no activity in cell-wall synthesis.

87. The answer is C. *(DiPalma, 3/e. pp 677–678. Gilman, 8/e. pp 972–973.)* Thiabendazole (Mintezol) has been shown to be effective against *Strongyloides*, cutaneous larva migrans, and *Trichuris*. Adverse effects consist of nausea, vertigo, headache, and weakness. Treatment usually involves oral administration for several days. It has been found to be ineffective in *Ascaris, N. americanus, E. vermicularis*, and *T. saginata*.

88. The answer is C. *(DiPalma, 3/e. pp 622–624. Gilman, 8/e. pp 1047–1057.)* Precipitation of sulfonamide crystals may form concentrations that injure the tubular epithelium or the epithelium of the pelvis of the kidney and obstruct the flow of urine. The crystallization is more frequently observed if the solubility of the drug in the urine is low, the pH of the urine is low, or the concentration of the drug in the urine is high. Simultaneous administration of several sulfonamides, each at less than half its normal concentration, permits an adequate bacteriostatic blood concentration to be reached without the risk of renal damage independent of the route of administration.

89. The answer is E. *(DiPalma, 3/e. pp 649, 657. Gilman, 8/e. p 955.)* Strains of *P. falciparum* that are sensitive to chloroquine are treated with chloroquine as the drug of choice. Chloroquine can be used for both prophylaxis and treatment of uncomplicated attacks. It can be administered parenterally as well as orally.

90. The answer is E. *(DiPalma, 3/e. pp 641–642. Gilman, 8/e. pp 1184–1186.)* Acyclovir is a nucleoside analogue of the pyrimidine guanosine. The mechanism of activity involves its conversion to a triphosphate and subsequent inhibition of synthesis of viral DNA. Its activity is highly selective. Acyclovir is available for topical, oral, and intravenous administration and is highly effective against herpes simplex, varicella-zoster, and Epstein-Barr viruses.

91. The answer is C. *(DiPalma, 3/e. p 616. Gilman, 8/e. pp 1127–1129.)* Hematologic toxicity is by far the most important adverse effect of chloramphenicol. The toxicity consists of two types: bone marrow depression (common) and aplastic anemia (rare). Chloramphenicol can produce a potentially fatal toxic reaction, the gray baby syndrome, caused by diminished ability of neonates to conjugate chloramphenicol with resultant high serum concentrations. Tetracyclines produce staining of the teeth and phototoxicity.

92. The answer is D. *(DiPalma, 3/e. pp 447, 660. Gilman, 8/e. pp 1011–1013.)* Both trimethoprim-sulfamethoxazole and pentamidine are effective in pneumonia caused by *P. carinii*. This protozoal disease usually occurs in immunodeficient patients such as those with AIDS. Nifurtimox is effective in trypanosomiasis and metronidazole in amebiasis and leishmaniasis, as well as in anaerobic bacterial infections. Penicillins are not considered drugs of choice for this particular disease state.

93. The answer is B. *(DiPalma, 3/e. p 594. Gilman, 8/e. pp 1085–1092.)* The cephalosporins are generally divided into three major categories that have been labeled first, second, and third generations. The cephalosporins are listed in one of these categories according to the spectrum of activity. The first generation includes cephalexin, cephalothin, cefazolin, cephradine, and cephapirin; the second generation cefamandole and cefoxitin; and the third generation cefoperazone, cefotaxime, and moxalactam.

94. The answer is D. *(DiPalma, 3/e. p 658. Gilman, 8/e. pp 1002–1005.)* Metronidazole is not preferred for use against asymptomatic carriers of cysts because it is rapidly absorbed from the intestine; luminal drugs, such as iodoquinol or diloxanide furoate, are preferred, either alone or in combination with metronidazole. Metronidazole is much less toxic than emetine, which had been frequently used in the past. Both the luminal and tissue stages of the ameba are susceptible to metronidazole.

95. The answer is B. *(DiPalma, 3/e. pp 608–611. Gilman, 8/e. pp 1098–1113.)* Aminoglycosides are combined with other antibiotics to increase their antibiotic activity (synergy) and also to decrease the emergence of resistant organisms, especially gram-negative organisms. Generally the combination of two differently acting antibiotics increases the antimicrobial spectrum. The ability of the aminoglycosides to be absorbed orally is not enhanced by combination with other antibiotics nor are there any significant drug interactions or a decrease in potential systemic toxicities.

96. The answer is A. *(DiPalma, 3/e. p 612. Gilman, 8/e. pp 1112–1113.)* Streptomycin, colistin, lincomycin, and clindamycin—in addition to neomycin listed in the question—have also been demonstrated to exert neuromuscular blocking effects that are synergistic with competitive blocking agents such as ether or tubocurarine. This effect is of clinical importance when these antibiotics are administered in large doses intravenously or intraperitoneally.

97. The answer is A. *(DiPalma, 3/e. p 617. Gilman, 8/e. pp 1125–1130.)* Chloramphenicol is the drug of choice in symptomatic *Salmonella* infection (typhoid fever) and also in *Haemophilus influenzae* meningitis in small children, especially when the strain is resistant to ampicillin. Tetracyclines are the drugs of choice for the treatment of brucellosis and cholera. Chloramphenicol may be used in the treatment of brucellosis, however, if tetracycline is contraindicated. Ordinary urinary tract infection and pharyngitis should be treated initially with penicillin.

98. The answer is C. *(DiPalma, 3/e. pp 592–595. Gilman, 8/e. pp 1085–1092.)* Both cephalosporins and penicillins contain a β-lactam ring, and both drugs are sensitive to inactivation by β-lactamase to varying degrees. The mechanisms of action of the two antibiotics are similar: cross-linking of D-alanyl-D-alanine of the peptidoglycan in the formation of bacterial cell walls is inhibited. Cross-allergenicity presumably occurs on the basis of hypersensitivity to similar breakdown products. The majority of the cephalosporins are administered parenterally.

99. The answer is A. *(DiPalma, 3/e. pp 612–613. Gilman, 8/e. pp 1098–1113.)* All the aminoglycosides are potentially toxic to both branches of the eighth cranial nerve. The evidence indicates that the sensory receptor portions of the inner ear are affected rather than the nerve itself. Nephrotoxicity may develop during or after the use of an aminoglycoside. It is generally more common in the elderly when there is preexisting renal dysfunction. In most patients renal function gradually improves after discontinuation of therapy. Aminoglycosides rarely cause neuromuscular blockade that can lead to progressive flaccid paralysis and potential fatal respiratory arrest. Hypersensitivity and dermatologic reactions occasionally occur following use of aminoglycosides.

100. The answer is B. *(DiPalma, 3/e. pp 634–636. Gilman, 8/e. pp 1165–1168.)* Amphotericin B is poorly absorbed from the gastrointestinal tract. The agent's antifungal activity is contingent upon binding of the drug to a sterol moiety present in the membranes of sensitive fungi, which changes the membranes' permeability. Over 80 percent of patients given amphotericin B develop decreased renal function and abnormal urinary sediments. The side effects can be so serious that amphotericin B is restricted to the treatment of severe systemic fungal infections.

101. The answer is B. *(DiPalma, 3/e. p 616. Gilman, 8/e. pp 1125–1130.)* The often fatal gray baby syndrome of chloramphenicol toxicity consists of abdominal distention; vasomotor collapse; diarrhea; rapid, irregular respirations progressing to flaccidity; ashen-gray color (owing to pallid cyanosis); and hypothermia. It is related to the failure of chloramphenicol to be conjugated with glucuronic acid. Neonates have insufficient glucuronyltransferase for conjugation and inadequately developed renal mechanisms for effective excretion of the unconjugated drug.

102. The answer is B. *(DiPalma, 3/e. pp 621–623. Gilman, 8/e. pp 1047–1057.)* The mechanism of action of sulfonamides is thought to be through competitive antagonism of *p*-aminobenzoic acid, the utilization of which by bacteria is essential to synthesis of folic acid. An excess of folic or *p*-aminobenzoic acid will overcome the bacteriostatic effect of sulfonamides. Bacteria that do not need folic acid or can use preformed folic acid are not affected by sulfonamides. Methotrexate inhibits folic acid production and would not interfere with the sulfonamide antimicrobial activity.

103. The answer is B. *(DiPalma, 3/e. p 621. Gilman, 8/e. pp 1054–1057, 1118, 1173.)* The diaminopyrimidines trimethoprim and pyrimethamine are selective inhibitors of dihydrofolate reductase; they have less of an effect on dihydrofolate reductase obtained from mammalian sources. The combination of a diaminopyrimidine and a sulfonamide is synergistic. The combination of trimethoprim and sulfamethoxazole results in the inhibition of the activity of dihydrofolate reductase by trimethoprim and in the inhibition of bacterial synthesis of dihydrofolic acid by the competition between *p*-aminobenzoic acid and sulfamethoxazole. Tetracycline inhibits the production of bacterial proteins, and griseofulvin interferes with synthesis of nucleic acid.

104–107. The answers are: 104-A, 105-C, 106-E, 107-F. *(DiPalma, 3/e. pp 580–581, 602, 609, 615. Katzung, 4/e. pp 545–552.)* Bacterial cells differ from mammalian cells in having a rigid cell wall, which actually forms a compression jacket. The internal osmotic pressure is very high and damage to the cell wall results in bursting of the bacterium. Cephalosporins, penicillins, vancomycin, and ristocetin all inhibit cell-wall synthesis. In particular, penicillins and cephalosporins block the final step in cell-wall synthesis by inhibiting transpeptidase enzymes.

Chloramphenicol, erythromycin, lincomycin, tetracyclines, and aminoglycoside antibiotics such as amikacin, gentamicin, kanamycin, neomycin, and streptomycin exert their antibacterial action through inhibition of protein synthesis. Erythromycin inhibits binding of aminoacyl tRNAs to the 50S ribosome subunit. Aminoglycosides bind to the 30S subunit as does tetracycline.

Other antibiotics—such as amphotericin B, colistin, nystatin, and polymyxins—inhibit bacteria by disrupting the cellular membrane.

108–112. The answers are: 108-C, 109-G, 110-A, 111-I, 112-E. *(Katzung, 4/e. pp 666–680.)* Pinworm infestation should be treated with pyrantel in conjunction with rigid standards of personal hygiene. Pyrantel is also the drug of choice against *Ascaris lumbricoides*. A single dose of 11 mg/kg, to a maximum of 1 g, is sufficient.

Filariasis is effectively treated with diethylcarbamazine, a piperazine derivative, which both suppresses and, in most cases, cures the infection. The drug is inactive against *Wuchereria bancrofti* in vitro. However, in vivo activity appears to be due to a sensitization of the microfilaria to phagocytosis by the fixed macrophages of the reticuloendothelial system.

Niclosamide is the agent of choice for treatment of *Taenia saginata* infections. It is highly effective and relatively free of side effects. These properties have resulted in its replacement of quinacrine, which has become obsolete.

Schistosomiasis responds well to antimony-containing compounds and niridazole. However, infection with *Schistosoma haematobium* responds best to praziquantel. A single oral dose of 40 mg/kg is sufficient.

Bithionol has been found useful in the treatment of infection by the sheep liver fluke *Fasciola hepatica* and the lung fluke *Paragonimus kellicotti*. Treatment usually involves the oral administration of 40 to 50 mg/kg, in divided doses on alternate days, for a total of 10 to 15 doses. Chloroquine in large doses has also been successful in the therapy of infection by lung flukes.

113–117. The answers are: 113-F, 114-A, 115-C, 116-E, 117-H. *(DiPalma, 3/e. pp 583–591. Katzung, 4/e. pp 553–558.)* Because of its long duration of action, benzathine penicillin G is given as a single injection of 1.2 million units intramuscularly every 3 or 4 weeks for the treatment of syphilis. This persistence of action reduces the need for repeated injections, costs, and local trauma. Benzathine penicillin G is also administered for group A, beta-hemolytic streptococcal pharyngitis and pyoderma.

Methicillin is a β-lactamase-resistant (penicillinase-resistant) penicillin that is acid-labile but must be administered by the parenteral route. It is effective against nearly all strains of *Staphylococcus aureus*. Methicillin is much more effective against penicillinase-producing strains than is penicillin G.

Piperacillin along with mezlocillin and azlocillin is commonly referred to as an extended-spectrum penicillin because of its broad spectrum of activity. It is particularly effective against *Klebsiella* and *Pseudomonas*. Piperacillin is available as a powder for solubilization and injection.

Amoxicillin is closely related to ampicillin but is better tolerated and has better absorption in the gastrointestinal tract with fewer gastrointestinal side effects. Amoxicillin's spectrum of activity is identical to that of ampicillin, except that ampicillin appears to be more effective against *Shigellosis*.

Carbenicillin is an effective penicillin for the treatment of *Pseudomonas* and *Proteus* infections. It is generally given by the intravenous route but contains 4.7 meq of sodium per gram, which may under chronic use cause an elevation of serum sodium levels. Large doses are often necessary.

Cancer Chemotherapy and Immunology

The Cell Cycle
- Effect of various chemotherapeutic agents on different stages of the cell cycle
- General toxicities of chemotherapeutic agents on normal tissues

Alkylating Agents
- Nitrogen mustards
  - Mechlorethamine HCl*
  - Chlorambucil
  - Melphalan
  - Ifosfamide
  - Cyclophosphamide
  - Uracil mustard
- Nitrosoureas
  - Lomustine*
  - Carmustine
  - Streptozocin
- Miscellaneous
  - Thiotepa
  - Busulfan
  - Pipobroman
  - Cisplatin*
  - Carboplatin

Antimetabolites
- Methotrexate, trimetrexate
- Mercaptopurine, thioguanine
- Fluorouracil and floxuridine
- Cytabarine

Hormones
- Androgens
  - Testolactone*
- Antiandrogen
  - Flutamide*
- Progestins
  - Megestrol acetate*
  - Medroxyprogesterone acetate
- Estrogens
  - Diethylstilbestrol diphosphate*
  - Polyestradiol phosphate
- Estrogen/nitrogen mustard
  - Estramustine phosphate sodium
- Antiestrogen
  - Tamoxifen citrate*
- Gonadotropin-releasing hormone analogue
  - Leuprolide acetate*
  - Goserelin acetate

Antibiotics
- Bleomycin sulfate*
- Anthracyclines
  - Idarubicin HCl
  - Doxorubicin HCl*
  - Daunorubicin HCl
  - Mitoxantrone HCl
- Mitomycin*
- Dactinomycin
- Plicamycin

Mitotic Inhibitors
- Etoposide
- Vincristine sulfate*
- Vinblastine sulfate

Miscellaneous
- Interferon alfa-2a, alfa-2b, alpha-n3*
- Levamisole HCl*
- Altretamine
- Hydroxyurea
- BCG intravesical
- Procarbazine HCl

Decarbazine
Mitotane
Asparaginase*
Radiopharmaceuticals
Sodium iodide ^{131}I*
Sodium phosphate ^{32}P
Immunopharmacologic Drugs
Cytotoxic
Azathioprine*
Cyclophosphamide
Vincristine
Methotrexate
Cytarabine
Specific T-cell inhibitor
Cyclosporine*
Hormonal
Prednisone*
Other corticosteroids
Antibodies
Antilymphocyte globulin (ALG)
Muromonab-CD_3
$Rh_o(D)$ immune globulin

DIRECTIONS: Each question below contains five suggested responses. Select the **one best** response to each question.

118. A 32-year-old cancer patient, who has smoked two packs of cigarettes a day for 10 years, presents a decreased pulmonary function test. Physical examination and chest x-rays suggest preexisting pulmonary disease. All the following drugs may be prescribed EXCEPT

(A) vinblastine (Velban)
(B) doxorubicin (Adriamycin)
(C) mithramycin (Mitracin)
(D) bleomycin (Blenoxane)
(E) *cis*-diamminedichloroplatinum (Platinol)

119. The most effective drug for immunosuppression of rejection of the allografted kidney is

(A) azathioprine
(B) cyclosporine
(C) 5-fluorouracil
(D) cyclophosphamide
(E) vincristine

120. Which phase of the cell cycle is primarily affected by antimetabolite chemotherapeutic agents?

(A) Growth 1 (G_1) phase
(B) Growth 2 (G_2) phase
(C) Mitosis (M) phase
(D) Synthesis (S) phase
(E) Growth 0 (G_0) phase (resting)

121. The tumor LEAST susceptible to "cell cycle–specific" anticancer agents is

(A) acute lymphoblastic leukemia
(B) acute granulocytic leukemia
(C) Burkitt's lymphoma
(D) adenocarcinoma of the colon
(E) choriocarcinoma

122. All the following are cell cycle–specific (CCS) agents EXCEPT

(A) mercaptopurine
(B) fluorouracil
(C) bleomycin
(D) busulfan
(E) vincristine

123. A nucleophilic attack on DNA that causes the disruption of base pairing occurs as a result of administration of

(A) cyclophosphamide
(B) fluorouracil
(C) methotrexate
(D) prednisone
(E) thioguanine

124. The antineoplastic chemotherapeutic agent that is classified as an alkylating agent is

(A) thioguanine
(B) busulfan
(C) bleomycin
(D) vincristine
(E) tamoxifen

125. All the following statements regarding the chemotherapy of cancer are true EXCEPT

(A) 50 percent of all newly diagnosed cancer patients will be cured of their disease
(B) chemotherapy is the only treatment that can effectively treat systemic disease
(C) chemotherapy only kills cancer cells and not normal dividing cells
(D) chemotherapy possesses numerous side effects, such as nausea, vomiting, and suppression of bone marrow
(E) new agents are cell cycle–specific

126. Which of the following is a chemotherapeutic drug that possesses a mechanism of action involving alkylation?

(A) Cyclophosphamide
(B) Methotrexate
(C) Tamoxifen
(D) Fluorouracil
(E) Bleomycin

127. Which one of the following statements is correct about antimetabolites?

(A) They are structural analogues of naturally occurring substances
(B) They are nontoxic
(C) They do not interfere with metabolic processes
(D) Procarbazine is an example
(E) They have little or no effect on cell proliferation

128. All the following drugs are used in the MOPP protocol for the treatment of Hodgkin's disease EXCEPT

(A) prednisone
(B) vincristine
(C) procarbazine
(D) methotrexate
(E) mechlorethamine

129. All the following statements concerning alkylating agents are true EXCEPT

(A) they are able to form covalent bonds with nucleophilic sites on nucleic acids
(B) they possess little or no toxicity in the host
(C) they are cytotoxic owing to their activity against DNA
(D) they are able to form a positive carbonium ion
(E) they can affect any part of the cell cycle

130. Cardiotoxicity limits the clinical usefulness of which one of the following antitumor antibiotics?

(A) Dactinomycin (Cosmegen)
(B) Doxorubicin (Adriamycin)
(C) Bleomycin (Blenoxane)
(D) Cisplatin
(E) Vincristine

131. All the following drugs are considered to be cell cycle–specific EXCEPT

(A) 5-fluorouracil
(B) methotrexate
(C) 6-mercaptopurine
(D) vincristine
(E) tamoxifen

132. All the following are true statements regarding allopurinol EXCEPT

(A) it inhibits the metabolism of 6-mercaptopurine
(B) it increases the antineoplastic action of 6-mercaptopurine
(C) it inhibits xanthine oxidase
(D) it decreases serum uric acid levels
(E) it possesses uricosuric activity

133. All the following statements are true concerning cyclosporines EXCEPT

(A) they cross cell membranes easily
(B) they bind to a family of intracellular proteins called *cyclophilins*
(C) they inhibit the production of interleukin 2 (IL-2) by helper T cells
(D) they are cytotoxic and depress bone marrow
(E) active biotransformation of cyclosporine is by cytochrome P-450

134. Azathioprine is correctly characterized by all the following statements EXCEPT

(A) it is a prodrug
(B) it has little action on an established graft rejection
(C) it is poorly absorbed in the GI tract
(D) it has a nonselective action in the suppression of lymphoid cells
(E) it greatly increases the susceptibility of the patient to intercurrent infections

135. A correct statement about methotrexate is that it

(A) binds to sites on the enzyme dihydrofolate reductase
(B) is indicated in lung cancer
(C) is indicated in colon cancer
(D) is classified as an alkylating agent
(E) is classified as an antibiotic agent

136. Glucocorticoids perform all the following immunosuppressive actions EXCEPT

(A) decrease the concentration of antibodies in the circulation
(B) inhibit the synthesis of prostaglandins and leukotrienes
(C) lyse T cells
(D) increase catabolism of gamma G globulin (IgG) on continuous administration
(E) diminish the ability to withstand infections and heal wounds

137. Which of the following is considered to be the effective mechanism of action of the vinca alkaloids?

(A) Inhibition of the function of microtubules
(B) Damage and prevention of repair of DNA
(C) Inhibition of DNA synthesis
(D) Inhibition of protein synthesis
(E) Inhibition of purine synthesis

DIRECTIONS: Each group of questions below consists of lettered headings followed by a set of numbered items. For each numbered item select the **one** lettered heading with which it is **most** closely associated. Each lettered heading may be used **once, more than once, or not at all.**

Questions 138–142

For each of the drugs below, select the characteristic with which it is most likely to be associated.

(A) Used in treatment of Hodgkin's lymphoma
(B) Classified as an alkylating agent and orally administered
(C) Retained specifically in beta cells of the islets of Langerhans
(D) Used as a single agent against malignant melanoma
(E) Classified as an antitumor antibiotic and results in a high incidence of bone marrow suppression
(F) Used in treatment of breast cancer
(G) Classified as a vinca alkaloid
(H) Used in malignant hypercalcemia
(I) Used in hairy cell leukemia
(J) Derived from hydrazine

138. Streptozotocin

139. Dacarbazine

140. Mitomycin

141. Mechlorethamine

142. Lomustine

Questions 143–147

For each of the drugs below, select the adverse reaction with which it is most closely associated.

(A) Aseptic hemorrhagic cystitis
(B) Cardiotoxicity
(C) Nephrotoxicity
(D) Oral and GI ulceration
(E) Exfoliative dermatitis
(F) Peripheral neuropathy
(G) Convulsions
(H) Pancreatitis
(I) Coma

143. Fluorouracil

144. Asparaginase

145. Cyclophosphamide (Cytoxan)

146. *cis*-Diamminedichloroplatinum (Platinol)

147. Procarbazine (Matulane)

Questions 148–152

For each of the chemotherapeutic agents below, choose the neoplasm against which it is most likely to be effective.

(A) Carcinoma of the breast
(B) Hairy cell leukemia
(C) Macroglobulinemia
(D) Prostate cancer
(E) Carcinoma of the thyroid
(F) Lung cancer
(G) Melanoma
(H) Hodgkin's disease
(I) Carcinoma of the colon
(J) Acute leukemia

148. Chlorambucil

149. Fluorouracil

150. Dacarbazine

151. Tamoxifen

152. Radioactive iodine (^{131}I)

Cancer Chemotherapy and Immunology

Answers

118. The answer is D. *(AMA Drug Evaluations Annual 1991, 7/e. pp 1174–1175. DiPalma, 3/e. pp 561–562.)* The potential serious adverse effect of bleomycin is pneumonitis and pulmonary fibrosis. This adverse effect appears to be both age- and dose-related. The clinical onset is characterized by decreasing pulmonary function, fine rales, cough, and diffuse basilar infiltrates. This complication develops in approximately 5 to 10 percent of patients treated with bleomycin. Thus, extreme caution must be used in patients with a preexisting history of pulmonary disease. All the other drugs listed in the question are effective against carcinomas and have not been associated with significant lung toxicity.

119. The answer is B. *(DiPalma, 3/e. pp 567–571. Gilman, 8/e. pp 1270, 1586.)* Cyclosporine is the preferred agent because it is a specific T-cell inhibitor and its success rate in protecting against rejection is considerably better than that of any other agent. All the other agents in the question are cytotoxic. Because of the severe adverse reactions with cyclosporine, it is used in conjunction with azathioprine, which reduces the required dose. Prednisone is also used in conjunction with cyclosporine.

120. The answer is D. *(DiPalma, 3/e. pp 549–551. Gilman, 8/e. p 1224.)* Antimetabolites such as methotrexate or 6-mercaptopurine inhibit DNA synthesis and thus act on the S phase. This phase of cell growth is preparatory to the second growth phase, which involves the production of specialized proteins necessary for mitosis of the cell. Steroid hormones act on the G_1 phase; antibiotics on the G_2 phase; plant alkaloids on the M phase; and alkylating agents are cell-cycle nonspecific.

121. The answer is D. *(DiPalma, 3/e. pp 549–551. Gilman, 8/e. pp 1202–1207.)* "Cell cycle–specific" cytotoxic agents are most effective in malignancies in which a large portion of the population of malignant cells is undergoing mitosis. In leukemia, lymphoma, choriocarcinoma, and other rapidly growing tumors, these agents may induce a high-percentage cell kill of the entire tumor and at least of those cells that are actively dividing. In slowly growing, solid tumors, such as carcinomas of the colon, the frequency of actively dividing cells is low, and perhaps the resting cells survive the cycle-specific agents and then can be recruited back into the proliferative cycle.

122. The answer is D. *(DiPalma, 3/e. pp 549–551. Gilman, 8/e. p 1220.)* Cell cycle–specific agents such as mercaptopurine, fluorouracil, bleomycin, and vincristine have proved to be the most effective against proliferating cells. Busulfan is an alkylating agent that binds to DNA and causes damage to these macromolecules. It is useful against low-growth as well as high-growth tumors and is classified as a cell cycle–nonspecific agent.

123. The answer is A. *(DiPalma, 3/e. pp 557–559. Gilman, 8/e. p 1210.)* Cyclophosphamide (Cytoxan), an alkylating agent, reacts with purine and pyrimidine bases of DNA to form bridges and dimers. These products interfere with DNA replication. 5-Fluorouracil, methotrexate, and 6-thioguanine are antimetabolites, and the steroid prednisone has some tumor-suppressive effects.

124. The answer is B. *(DiPalma, 3/e. p 552. Gilman, 8/e. pp 1205–1207, 1220.)* Busulfan is an alkylating agent that, in contrast to other alkylators, is an alkylsulfonate. Thioguanine is a purine antimetabolite. Bleomycin is classified as a chemotherapeutic antibiotic and vincristine is a vinca alkaloid. Tamoxifen is an antiestrogen hormone.

125. The answer is C. *(DiPalma, 3/e. pp 549–550. Katzung, 4/e. pp 683–686.)* Cancer chemotherapy, even with the best and most efficient detection procedures, can cure only approximately 50 percent of all newly diagnosed cancer patients. The reason for failure to cure is not delay in diagnosis. Surgery, chemotherapy, and radiation constitute the three forms of treatment for cancer, but only chemotherapy can effectively treat systemic disease. Both normal and cancerous dividing cells are killed by chemotherapy, which is one of its major drawbacks. Other serious side effects include nausea, vomiting, and suppression of bone marrow. The newer agents are specifically designed for their specific effects on the cell cycle.

126. The answer is A. *(DiPalma, 3/e. pp 557–560. Gilman, 8/e. pp 1205–1207.)* Cyclophosphamide is classified as a polyfunctional alkylating drug that transfers its alkyl groups to cellular components. The cytotoxic effect of this agent is directly associated with the alkylation of components of DNA. Methotrexate and fluorouracil are classified as antimetabolites that block intermediary metabolism to inhibit cell proliferation. Tamoxifen is an antiestrogen compound. Bleomycin is classified as an antibiotic chemotherapeutic agent.

127. The answer is A. *(DiPalma, 3/e. pp 551–552. Katzung, 4/e. pp 691–693.)* Antimetabolites are structural analogues of naturally occurring substances. They interfere with various metabolic processes and disrupt cell function and proliferation. These drugs may act in two ways: (1) by incorporation into the metabolic pathway and formation of a false metabolite that is nonfunctional, or (2) by inhibition of the catalytic function of an enzyme or enzyme system. Procarbazine is classified not as an antimetabolite but as an alkylating agent.

128. The answer is D. *(DiPalma, 3/e. pp 560, 563, 564. Katzung, 4/e. p 706.)* The drugs used in the MOPP regimen include mechlorethamine (Mustargen), vincristine (Oncovin), procarbazine (Matulane), and prednisone. Mechlorethamine is given intravenously and may cause nausea and vomiting. Vincristine is also given intravenously and is associated with adverse effects that include hair loss and neuromuscular disturbances. Procarbazine and prednisone are given orally. The administration of this combination of drugs in a defined cyclical schedule is the treatment of choice for stages III and IV of Hodgkin's disease and can be curative. The MOPP regimen is the standard against which other combination drug protocols for the treatment of Hodgkin's disease are measured.

129. The answer is B. *(DiPalma, 3/e. p 557. Gilman, 8/e. pp 1213–1214.)* The alkylating agents are highly reactive compounds with the ability to form covalent bonds with nucleophilic sites on molecules such as nucleic acids. This is usually accomplished through the formation of a positively charged carbonium ion. The cytotoxic effects of these agents most likely reflect their ability to bind to the nucleotides of DNA. The alkylators have an effect during any part of the cell cycle (cell cycle–nonspecific). Because of their nonspecificity, these compounds produce a significant number of adverse effects in the host.

130. The answer is B. *(DiPalma, 3/e. pp 561–562. Gilman, 8/e. pp 1238–1239, 1250.)* Dactinomycin's major toxicities include stomatitis, alopecia, and bone marrow depression. Bleomycin's toxicities include edema of the hands, alopecia, and stomatitis. Cisplatin produces both nephrotoxicity and ototoxicity. The clinical toxicity of vincristine is mostly neurologic. Doxorubicin causes cardiotoxicity as well as alopecia and bone marrow depression. The cardiotoxicity has been linked to a lipid peroxidation within cardiac cells.

131. The answer is E. *(DiPalma, 3/e. pp 549–551. Gilman, 8/e. pp 1207–1208.)* Cell cycle–specific drugs inhibit growth at some phase in the growth cycle. These phases are classified as follows: G_1, a presynthetic phase; S, the DNA synthesis phase; G_2, the interval following the end of DNA synthesis;

and M, the mitosis phase during which the G_2 cell divides into two G_1 daughter cells. Purine synthesis is inhibited by 6-mercaptopurine and by methotrexate; deoxythymidine monophosphate synthesis is blocked by 5-fluorouracil. Each of these three drugs affects the S phase of cell growth. Vincristine, however, blocks the cell cycle at the mitotic phase. Tamoxifen is an antiestrogenic drug used for breast cancer.

132. The answer is E. *(DiPalma, 3/e. pp 555–556.)* Allopurinol is a very effective inhibitor of the enzyme that metabolizes xanthine and hypoxanthine to form uric acid. This enzyme, xanthine oxidase, also is responsible for the oxidation of 6-mercaptopurine. Allopurinol, by blocking this reaction, increases the exposure time of tumor cells to 6-mercaptopurine. In addition, through the same mechanism the production of uric acid will decrease in the serum but there is no increase in uric acid levels in the urine.

133. The answer is D. *(DiPalma, 3/e. pp 569–571. Gilman, 8/e. pp 1267–1270.)* Cyclosporine is not cytotoxic in the ordinary sense and hence does not depress bone marrow. This makes it suitable for immunosuppression in bone marrow transplants. Despite its large molecular size it crosses cell membranes easily and binds to a cytoplasmic protein known as cyclophilin. It selectively inhibits the activation of T cells. The production of IL-2 is greatly reduced by the action of cyclosporine on helper T cells. The ring structure of cyclosporine is resistant to cell attack, but the side chains are oxidized by the cytochrome P-450 liver enzyme system. Excretion is mainly via the bile and little cyclosporine appears in the urine.

134. The answer is C. *(DiPalma, 3/e. pp 566–569. Gilman, 8/e. pp 1270–1271.)* Azathioprine is converted in the body to mercaptopurine. It is well absorbed in the GI tract and this is the main avenue of administration. As a cytotoxic drug it suppresses all cells and especially rapidly growing ones. Thus the bone marrow and the GI mucosa are growth-inhibited. This gives rise to the GI symptoms and the increased incidence of infections. Late toxicity includes the increased risk of malignancy, especially skin cancers and lymphoid tumors.

135. The answer is A. *(DiPalma, 3/e. pp 552–554. Gilman, 8/e. pp 1226–1227.)* The principal action of methotrexate is to compete with folic acid for the active binding sites on the enzyme dihydrofolate reductase. Methotrexate is well absorbed from the GI tract and may be given intravenously or intramuscularly. It is indicated in acute lymphatic leukemia, choriocarcinoma, non-Hodgkin's lymphoma, mycosis fungoides, sarcoma of the bone, and cancer of the neck and head. It is classified as an antimetabolite along with trimetrexate, which is a close chemical relative.

136. The answer is A. *(DiPalma, 3/e. p 572. Gilman, 8/e. pp 1443–1445.)* Glucocorticoids do not significantly diminish the concentration of antibodies in the circulation. Rather their action concerns the B- and T-cell function of producing immune substances and leukotrienes. Their anti-inflammatory actions are probably related to the inhibition of the synthesis of prostaglandins. As sole agents they are not capable of preventing graft rejection but they are useful in conjunction with azathioprine and cyclosporine.

137. The answer is A. *(DiPalma, 3/e. p 562. Gilman, 8/e. pp 1208, 1237.)* The vinca alkaloids vincristine and vinblastine have proved valuable because they work on a different principle from most cancer chemotherapeutic agents. They (like colchicine) inhibit mitosis in metaphase by their ability to bind to tubulin. This prevents the formation of tubules and consequently the orderly arrangement of chromosomes, which apparently causes cell death.

138–142. The answers are: 138-C, 139-D, 140-E, 141-A, 142-B. *(DiPalma, 3/e. pp 549–564. Gilman, 8/e. pp 1206–1207.)* Streptozotocin is a nitrosourea-like antibiotic that contains a glucosamine moiety that allows it to be selectively taken up by the beta cells of the islets of Langerhans. Consequently, it appears to be useful in treating metastatic islet cell carcinoma.

Dacarbazine (DTIC) is a triazene derivative of alkylating agents that appears to require demethylation for activity. It has displayed significant antineoplastic action against malignant melanomas.

Mitomycin is a potent antibiotic that selectively inhibits DNA synthesis by its ability to alkylate and cross-link DNA. The drug causes a bone marrow suppression in up to 64 percent of patients.

Mechlorethamine, the first widely used anticancer agent, has been largely superseded by less toxic drugs. Nevertheless, this alkylating agent has an important role in the treatment of Hodgkin's lymphoma as a component in the chemotherapeutic regimen MOPP (mechlorethamine, vincristine [Oncovin], procarbazine, and prednisone).

Lomustine (CCNU) is a nitrosourea that is rapidly absorbed from the gastrointestinal tract and, thus, is orally active. The plasma half-life of this compound is quite short (less than 6 min). Because of their lipophilicity, the nitrosoureas, including CCNU, cross the blood-brain barrier and have been used to treat malignancies of the central nervous system.

143–147. The answers are: 143-D, 144-H, 145-A, 146-C, 147-F. *(DiPalma, 3/e. pp 548–565. Gilman, 8/e. pp 1205–1207.)* Aseptic hemorrhagic cystitis has been reported as an adverse reaction occurring in 5 to 10 percent of patients who receive cyclophosphamide (Cytoxan). This syndrome is usually reversible upon withdrawal of the drug; occurrence of this complication can be minimized by adequate fluid intake and frequent voiding.

The two major toxicities associated with *cis*-diamminedichloroplatinum (Platinol), a drug used in treating testicular tumors, are vomiting and nephrotoxicity. The focal acute necrosis observed in the kidney affects primarily the distal tubules and collecting ducts.

Procarbazine commonly produces a dose-related, reversible bone marrow depression including thrombocytopenia and leukopenia. Neurotoxicity is also associated with this drug in 10 to 20 percent of the patients receiving it. This is manifested as ataxia, disorders in consciousness, and peripheral neuropathies. Procarbazine may reduce plasma pyridoxal phosphate levels, a phenomenon that may be responsible for the neurotoxicity.

Fluorouracil is a pyrimidine antagonist that has a low neurotoxicity when compared with other fluorinated derivatives; however, its major toxicities are myelosuppression and oral or gastrointestinal ulceration. Leukopenia is the most frequent clinical manifestation of the myelosuppression.

Asparaginase is an enzyme that catalyzes the hydrolysis of serum asparagine to aspartic acid and ammonia. Major toxicities are related to antigenicity and pancreatitis. In addition, more than 50 percent of those treated present biochemical evidence of hepatic dysfunction.

148–152. The answers are: 148-C, 149-I, 150-G, 151-A, 152-E. *(DiPalma, 3/e. pp 548–565. Katzung, 4/e. pp 704–712.)* Chlorambucil is an alkylating agent that is administered orally. The drug causes moderate depression of peripheral blood counts and depression of bone marrow. Chlorambucil is, therefore, used for macroglobulinemia.

Fluorouracil (5-FU) is an antimetabolite that inhibits DNA synthesis. Cytotoxicity of 5-FU is mainly due to its effects on both DNA and RNA synthesis, and the drug is used systemically in the management of carcinomas of the head and neck and colon. Topically it is used for multiple actinic, or solar, keratoses.

Dacarbazine is a polyfunctional alkylating agent administered by the intravenous route with major toxicities of nausea, vomiting, and bone marrow depression. It is one of the current treatments of melanoma, with a response rate of about 20 percent. When used concurrently with other agents, dacarbazine has been reported to produce beneficial responses in Hodgkin's disease and various sarcomas.

Tamoxifen, an antiestrogenic compound, has been shown to be effective against breast cancer that is estrogen-sensitive. Tamoxifen is a competitive inhibitor of estrogen and binds to estrogen receptors of estrogen-sensitive tumors. Hot flashes, nausea, and vomiting are the most frequent adverse reactions and occur in 25 percent of patients.

Radioactive iodine (^{131}I) is an isotope that has significant activity in thyroid cancer and induces regression of tumors of a variety of histologic types (especially anaplastic types).

Cardiovascular System, Hematology, and Pulmonary System

Cardiac Glycosides
- Digoxin, digitoxin, deslanoside

Other Inotropic Agents
- Sympathomimetics
  - Epinephrine,* isoproterenol,* dopamine,* dobutamine
- Nonsympathomimetics
  - Theophylline,* amrinone,* milrinone

Vasodilators for Congestive Heart Failure
- Nitrates, sodium nitroprusside, captopril, enalapril, nifedipine

Antiarrhythmic Drugs
- 1A. Quinidine,* procainamide, disopyramide
- 1B. Lidocaine,* tocainide, mexiletine, phenytoin
- 1C. Flecainide,* encainide, propafenone
- 2. Propranolol (other beta blockers)
- 3. Amiodarone,* bretylium
- 4. Verapamil, diltiazem

Antianginal Drugs
- Nitrates and nitrites
  - Nitroglycerine,* amyl nitrite, pentaerythritol tetranitrate, isosorbide dinitrate
- Beta-adrenergic blocking drugs
  - (All members are useful; a good choice is the cardioselective ones such as acebutolol, atenolol, and metoprolol.)
- Calcium channel blockers
  - Nifedipine, verapamil, and diltiazem

Agents for hyperlipoproteinemia
- Bile acid sequestrants
- Colestipol, cholestyramine
- Nicotinic acid
- Clofibrate, gemfibrozil
- Probucol
- Lovastatin
- Dehydrothyroxine

Antihypertensive Drugs
- Thiazides
  - (All are effective; most commonly used are chlorothiazide and hydrochlorothiazide—see section on Diuretics)
- Sympatholytic agents
  - Centrally acting
    - Methyldopa, clonidine, guanabenz, guanfacine
  - Peripherally acting
    - Beta-adrenergic blocking agents
      - Propranolol, etc.
    - Alpha-adrenergic blocking agents
      - Prazosin, terazosin, reserpine, guanethidine, guanadrel
  - Arterial vasodilators
    - Hydralazine, minoxidil
- Angiotensin converting enzyme (ACE) inhibitors

Captopril, enalapril, lisinopril

Calcium channel blockers

Nifedipine, verapamil, diltiazem

Drugs for hypertensive emergencies

Trimethaphan, sodium nitroprusside, diazoxide, nifedipine, labetalol

Drugs for Chronic Obstructive Pulmonary Diseases (COPD)

Bronchodilators

Methylxanthines, theophylline, elixophyllin

Beta-receptor agonists

Epinephrine, isoproterenol, isoetharine, metaproterenol, terbutaline, albuterol

Anticholinergics

Atropine, ipratropium

Mediator-release inhibitors

Cromolyn sodium

Corticosteroids

Flunisolide, beclomethasone, triamcinolone

Hematologic Agents

Antianemia drugs

Iron-ferrous sulfate, vitamin B_{12}, folic acid

Iron detoxifiers, deferoxamine

Anticoagulant and procoagulant drugs

Heparin, oral anticoagulants

Warfarin and dicumarol

Inhibitors of platelet aggregation

Aspirin and NSAIDS

Fibrinolytic drugs, streptokinase, urokinase, tissue-type plasminogen activator t-PA (alteplase)

Procoagulant drugs

Systemic

Antihemophilic factor, factor VIII, factor IX complex, desmopressin, aminocaproic acid, tranexamic acid

Topical

Thrombin, absorbable gelatin, oxidized cellulose, microfibrillar collagen hemostat

DIRECTIONS: Each question below contains five suggested responses. Select the **one best** response to each question.

153. Dopamine is used as a pressor agent in cases of circulatory failure. All the following are cardiovascular effects of dopamine EXCEPT

(A) activation of $beta_1$ receptors in the heart
(B) increase in both systolic and, in higher doses, diastolic pressure
(C) activation of dopamine receptors in the splanchnic area
(D) reduction of renal blood flow
(E) activation of alpha receptors at higher doses

154. Amrinone is a useful inotropic agent in certain cases of heart failure. All the following are attributes of amrinone EXCEPT

(A) it has a bipyridine chemical structure
(B) it is used only intravenously
(C) it inhibits phosphodiesterase
(D) it causes peripheral vasodilation
(E) it decreases calcium inward flux

155. Which of the following is an antiarrhythmic agent that has relatively few electrophysiologic effects on normal myocardial tissue but suppresses the arrhythmogenic tendencies of ischemic myocardial tissues?

(A) Propranolol
(B) Procainamide
(C) Quinidine
(D) Lidocaine
(E) Disopyramide

156. Inhibitors of angiotensin converting enzyme must be used with caution in elderly persons because they are apt to cause

(A) skin rashes
(B) drug fever
(C) hepatic injury
(D) renal failure
(E) bone marrow depression

157. Caffeine and other methylxanthines useful in chronic obstructive pulmonary disease (COPD) have all the following pharmacologic actions EXCEPT

(A) increased secretion of acid and pepsin by the stomach
(B) constriction of central blood vessels
(C) relaxation of bronchial smooth muscle
(D) stimulation of cyclic AMP phosphodiesterase
(E) antagonism of adenosine receptors

158. Cromolyn has been found to be a useful drug in chronic obstructive pulmonary disease, especially asthma. It is believed to exert a beneficial effect because it is

(A) a bronchodilator
(B) an H_1 receptor blocker
(C) an anticholinergic
(D) an inhibitor of mediator release
(E) a $beta_2$ agonist

159. Which of the following drugs recommended for the lowering of blood cholesterol inhibits the synthesis of cholesterol by blocking 3-hydroxy-3-methylglutaryl–coenzyme A (HMG-CoA) reductase?

(A) Lovastatin
(B) Probucol
(C) Clofibrate
(D) Gemfibrozil
(E) Nicotinic acid

160. The ECG of a patient who is receiving digitalis in the therapeutic dose range would be likely to show

(A) prolongation of the QT interval
(B) prolongation of the PR interval
(C) symmetric peaking of the T wave
(D) widening of the QRS complex
(E) none of the above

161. A person is likely to be more susceptible to digitoxin toxicity if digitoxin is taken with which of the following drugs?

(A) Neomycin
(B) Hydrochlorothiazide
(C) Phenobarbital
(D) Thioridazine
(E) Estradiol

162. In a hypertensive patient who is taking insulin to treat diabetes, which of the following drugs is to be used with extra caution and advice to the patient?

(A) Hydralazine
(B) Prazosin (Minipress)
(C) Guanethidine (Ismelin)
(D) Propranolol (Inderal)
(E) Methyldopa (Aldomet)

163. Which of the following drugs is considered to be most effective in relieving and preventing ischemic episodes in patients with variant angina?

(A) Propranolol
(B) Nitroglycerine
(C) Sodium nitroprusside
(D) Nifedipine
(E) Isorbide dinitrate

164. The enhancement of contractility of the cardiac muscle fiber brought about by digitalis is related to

(A) increased cyclic AMP
(B) stimulation of calmodulin
(C) inhibition of the sodium pump
(D) beta-adrenergic stimulation
(E) increased production of adenosine

165. If both quinidine and digoxin are administered concurrently, which of the following effects does quinidine have on digoxin?

(A) The absorption of digoxin from the GI tract is decreased
(B) The metabolism of digoxin is prevented
(C) The concentration of digoxin in the plasma is increased
(D) The effect of digoxin on the AV node is antagonized
(E) The ability of digoxin to inhibit the Na^+,K^+-stimulated ATPase is reduced

166. Verapamil exerts its effects through which of the following actions?

(A) Preventing entry of calcium through slow channels
(B) Preventing depolarization of the cell membrane
(C) Increasing sodium entry
(D) Antagonizing the opening of the fast sodium channel
(E) Enhancing potassium efflux

167. All the following drugs may be used for the therapy of life-threatening hypertensive emergency (crisis) EXCEPT

(A) furosemide
(B) diazoxide
(C) nifedipine
(D) labetalol
(E) pindolol

168. Drugs that block the catecholamine uptake process—such as cocaine, tricyclic antidepressants, and phenothiazines—are apt to block the antihypertensive action of which of the following drugs?

(A) Propranolol
(B) Guanethidine
(C) Prazosin
(D) Hydralazine
(E) Diazoxide

169. Which of the following causes increased synthesis and secretion of aldosterone by the adrenal cortex?

(A) Renin
(B) Angiotensin I
(C) Angiotensin II
(D) Kallikrein
(E) Kininogen

170. Which of the following drugs does not cross the placenta and has no significant concentration in milk in the lactating female?

(A) Heparin
(B) Dicumarol
(C) Warfarin
(D) Phenindione
(E) Acenocoumarol

171. Which of the following antihypertensive drugs produces most of its effects by blocking alpha$_1$-adrenergic receptors in arterioles and venules?

(A) Pindolol
(B) Prazosin
(C) Minoxidil
(D) Phentolamine
(E) Clonidine

172. For the monotherapy of mild-to-moderate hypertension, all the following drugs would be suitable EXCEPT

(A) metoprolol
(B) minoxidil
(C) verapamil
(D) enalapril
(E) nifedipine

173. Nicotinic acid in the large doses used to treat hyperlipoproteinemia causes a cutaneous flush. The vasodilatory effect is due to

(A) release of histamine
(B) production of local prostaglandins
(C) release of platelet-derived growth factor (PDGF)
(D) production of nitric oxide (NO)
(E) calcium channel block

174. One type of hyperlipoproteinemia is characterized by elevated plasma levels of chylomicrons, normal plasma levels of β-lipoproteins, and the inability of any known drug to reduce lipoprotein levels. This is which of the following types of hyperlipoproteinemia?

(A) Type I
(B) Type IIa, IIb
(C) Type III
(D) Type IV
(E) Type V

175. Which of the following drugs would be indicated in a patient who still has heart failure after adequate therapy with diuretics and digoxin?

(A) Dobutamine
(B) Hydralazine
(C) Minoxidil
(D) Prazosin
(E) Enalapril

176. The antiarrhythmic drug tocainide has all the following pharmacologic actions EXCEPT

(A) sodium channel block
(B) local anesthetic action
(C) increased refractory period of the ventricle
(D) a long half-life of 10 to 12 h
(E) suppression of premature ventricular contractions

177. Angiotensin converting enzyme (ACE) inhibitors are associated with a high incidence of which of the following adverse reactions?

(A) Hepatitis
(B) Hypokalemia
(C) Agranulocytosis
(D) Proteinuria
(E) Hirsutism

178. Isoproterenol modifies the cardiovascular system by interaction mediated via which of the following receptors?

(A) $Beta_2$-adrenergic receptors in the heart
(B) $Alpha_1$-adrenergic receptors in arterioles
(C) $Beta_1$-adrenergic receptors in arterioles
(D) $Beta_2$-adrenergic receptors in arterioles
(E) $Alpha_2$-adrenergic receptors in the brain

179. Digitalis is given to patients with atrial fibrillation because it

(A) decreases the excitability of the atria
(B) increases conductivity in the AV node
(C) decreases automaticity of the atria
(D) increases the effective refractory period in the AV node
(E) has muscarinic effects

180. Nitroglycerine, a frequently used cardiovascular drug, has all the following actions EXCEPT

(A) it can cause adverse reactions of headache and tachycardia
(B) it undergoes significant first-pass biotransformation
(C) it is used for congestive heart failure
(D) it decreases total coronary blood flow
(E) it is converted to nitrite by the smooth muscle cell

181. Verapamil, a drug that may be used in place of digitalis to treat arrhythmias, is correctly characterized by all the following statements EXCEPT

(A) it possesses significant first-pass biotransformation following oral administration
(B) it can cause adverse reactions such as constipation and headaches
(C) it reduces calcium influx through voltage-dependent calcium channels
(D) it is useful in the management of supraventricular arrhythmias
(E) it is useful in the management of ventricular arrhythmias

182. True statements regarding the mechanism of action of the nitrites and organic nitrates in causing smooth muscle relaxation include all the following EXCEPT

(A) nitric oxide (NO) is formed
(B) adenyl cyclase is inhibited
(C) a cyclic GMP–dependent protein kinase is stimulated
(D) the light chain of myosin is dephosphorylated
(E) the mechanism is similar to that of endothelial-derived relaxing factor (EDRF)

183. All the following deficiencies or agents may cause megaloblastic anemia EXCEPT

(A) deficiency of folic acid
(B) methotrexate therapy for leukemia
(C) trimethoprim therapy
(D) phenytoin therapy for epilepsy
(E) L-dopa therapy of parkinsonism

184. Significant relaxation of smooth muscle of both venules and arterioles is produced by which of the following drugs?

(A) Hydralazine
(B) Minoxidil (Loniten)
(C) Diazoxide (Hyperstat)
(D) Sodium nitroprusside
(E) Nifedipine

185. Patients with genetically low levels of *N*-acetyltransferase are more prone to develop a lupus erythematosus–like syndrome with which of the following drugs?

(A) Propranolol (Inderal)
(B) Procainamide
(C) Digitoxin
(D) Captopril
(E) Quinidine

186. The automaticity of Purkinje's fibers of the heart can be increased by all the following EXCEPT

(A) epinephrine
(B) digitalis
(C) quinidine
(D) low concentrations of potassium
(E) isoproterenol

187. Beta-adrenergic blocking agents have a beneficial effect in angina because they do all the following EXCEPT

(A) slow the heart rate
(B) lower blood pressure
(C) buffer the heart against sympathetic stimulation
(D) cause peripheral vasodilation
(E) reduce myocardial contractility

188. The advantages inhibitors of angiotensin converting enzyme have in the therapy of congestive heart failure include all the following EXCEPT

(A) lack of renal toxicity
(B) no tendency to develop tolerance
(C) decrease in adrenal production of aldosterone
(D) reduction in both preload and afterload
(E) lowering of blood pressure

189. Which of the following anemias would be treated with cyanocobalamin (vitamin B_{12})?

(A) Anemia in infants who are undergoing rapid growth
(B) Anemia associated with chelosis, dysphagia, gastritis, and hypochlorhydria
(C) Anemia associated with small, bizarre cells poorly filled with hemoglobin
(D) Anemia associated with infestation by *Diphyllobothrium latum*
(E) Bleeding from a gastric ulcer

190. The preferred agent to combat extreme digitalis overdose is

(A) potassium
(B) calcium
(C) phenytoin
(D) Fab fragments of digitalis antibodies
(E) magnesium

191. The nitrates remain the most valuable agents for the therapy of angina pectoris. Valid statements with respect to their overall mechanism of action include all the following EXCEPT

(A) nitrates cause reflex tachycardia
(B) in normal subjects nitrates can induce a transient increase in total coronary flow by directly dilating coronary arteries
(C) in coronary artery disease beneficial actions of nitrates are attributable to a decreased myocardial oxygen requirement
(D) nitrates increase venous capacitance and thus cause a decrease in myocardial preload
(E) nitrates are incompatible with beta blockers

192. Calcium channel blocking drugs have gained wide prominence in recent years. They relate to the role of calcium in the control function of several organ systems. All the following may be altered therapeutically by restricting calcium influx EXCEPT

(A) vascular smooth muscle
(B) skeletal muscle
(C) cardiac muscle
(D) glandular secretion
(E) esophageal smooth muscle

193. Drugs that reduce the size of a preformed fibrin clot have recently proved to be especially useful. Agents capable of dissolving fibrin clots include all the following EXCEPT

(A) tissue plasminogen activator (tPA)
(B) urokinase
(C) streptokinase
(D) factor IX complex
(E) anistreplase (streptokinase-plasminogen complex)

194. Megaloblastic anemia may be responsive to administration of all the following EXCEPT

(A) cyanocobalamin
(B) intrinsic factor concentrate
(C) ferrous sulfate
(D) folic acid
(E) folinic acid

195. Endogenous heparin is characterized by all the following statements EXCEPT

(A) it is found largely in mast cells
(B) it is a sulfonated mucopolysaccharide
(C) it is inhibited by protamine sulfate
(D) it is able to release a lipemia-clearing factor
(E) it crosses the placental barrier

196. Precautions advisable when using lovastatin include

(A) serum transaminase measurements
(B) renal function studies
(C) acoustic measurements
(D) monthly complete blood counts
(E) avoidance of bile acid sequestrants

197. The drug of choice in treating an acute attack of reentrant supraventricular tachycardia is

(A) verapamil
(B) digitalis
(C) propranolol
(D) phenylephrine
(E) edrophonium

198. All the following statements concerning agents that block calcium influx are true EXCEPT

(A) nifedipine is more suitable than diltiazem in the presence of atrioventricular conduction abnormalities
(B) nifedipine causes less arteriolar dilation than verapamil or diltiazem
(C) in the presence of atrial tachycardia, flutter, or fibrillation, verapamil is a preferred drug
(D) heart failure is not a contraindication to any of the blockers of calcium influx
(E) concurrent use with beta-adrenergic blockers causes greater cardiac depression

DIRECTIONS: Each group of questions below consists of lettered headings followed by a set of numbered items. For each numbered item select the **one** lettered heading with which it is **most** closely associated. Each lettered heading may be used **once, more than once, or not at all.**

Questions 199–202

Listed below are drugs designed to lower blood cholesterol. For each of these drugs select the most appropriate mechanism of action.

(A) Inhibits lipolysis in adipose tissue
(B) Decreases cholesterol synthesis at a rate-limiting step
(C) Increases the excretion of bile acids
(D) Decreases esterification of triglycerides in the liver and increases the activity of lipoprotein lipase
(E) Increases the activity of the lipid-clearing factor of heparin

199. Cholestyramine (Questran)

200. Gemfibrozil (Lopid)

201. Lovastatin (Mevacor)

202. Nicotinic acid

Questions 203–207

Match each route of administration and treatment indication with the correct drug.

(A) Isoproterenol
(B) Terbutaline
(C) Nitroglycerine
(D) Cromolyn sodium
(E) Beclomethasone
(F) Sodium nitroprusside

203. Administered transdermally for angina pectoris

204. Administered parenterally to produce myocardial stimulation

205. Administered by aerosol for bronchial asthma

206. Administered intravenously for heart failure

207. Administered orally to produce bronchial dilatation

Questions 208–212

It is customary today to classify antiarrhythmic drugs according to their mechanism of action. This is best defined by intracellular recordings that yield monophasic action potentials. In the accompanying figure, the monophasic action potentials of (A) slow response fiber (SA node) and (B) fast Purkinje fiber are shown. For each description that follows, choose the appropriate drug with which the change in character of the monophasic action potential is likely to be associated.

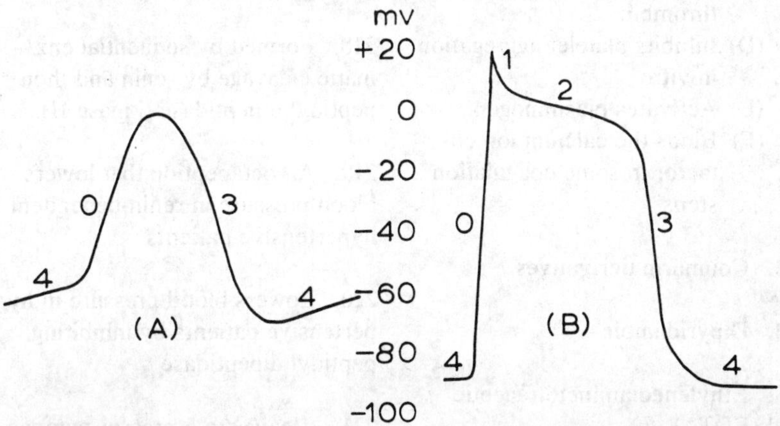

(A) Digitalis
(B) Amiodarone (Cordarone)
(C) Mexiletine (Mexitil)
(D) Nifedipine (Procardia)
(E) Propranolol (Inderal)
(F) Flecainide (Tambocor)
(G) Disopyramide (Norpace)
(H) Verapamil (Calan, Isoptin)

208. Moderate phase 0 depression and slow conduction; prolonged repolarization

209. Affects mainly phase 3 prolonging repolarization

210. Marked phase 0 depression and slow conduction; little effect on repolarization

211. Affects mainly phase 4 of the monophasic action potential of the atrium

212. Minimal phase 0 depression and little slowing of conduction; no effect on or shortens repolarization

Questions 213–217

Match the drugs below with the appropriate action.

(A) Raises the plasma level of factor IX
(B) Inhibits thrombin and early coagulation steps
(C) Inhibits synthesis of prothrombin
(D) Inhibits platelet aggregation in vitro
(E) Activates plasminogen
(F) Binds the calcium ion cofactor in some coagulation steps

213. Coumarin derivatives

214. Dipyridamole

215. Ethylenediaminetetraacetic acid (EDTA)

216. Heparin

217. Streptokinase

Questions 218–222

Match the descriptions below with the appropriate agent.

(A) Angiotensin I
(B) Angiotensin II
(C) Clonidine
(D) Saralasin
(E) Captopril

218. Formed by sequential enzymatic cleavage by renin and then peptidyl dipeptidase (kinase II)

219. An octapeptide that lowers blood pressure in renin-dependent hypertensive patients

220. Lowers blood pressure in hypertensive patients by inhibiting peptidyl dipeptidase

221. Cleaves to a pressor octapeptide on single passage through the lungs

222. An octapeptide that is a potent vasoconstrictor

Cardiovascular System, Hematology, and Pulmonary System

Answers

153. The answer is D. *(DiPalma, 3/e. pp 105, 358. Katzung, 4/e. p 100.)* Dopamine is the immediate metabolic precursor of norepinephrine. It has many of the attributes of this drug, such as activating at higher doses alpha receptors in the blood vessels and thus causing arteriolar vasoconstriction and a rise in blood pressure. It also activates $beta_1$ receptors in the heart. However, of major importance is the effect on special dopamine receptors in the splanchnic and renal vasculature. These cause vasodilation, and hence renal vascular tone is reduced and blood flow increased. This makes dopamine useful in some types of shock.

154. The answer is E. *(DiPalma, 3/e. pp 357–358. Katzung, 4/e. p 158.)* Amrinone, a bipyridine, differs in chemical structure from digitalis and catecholamines. Oral absorption is good, but amrinone has unacceptable toxicity by this route and so is used only intravenously. The mechanism of action is unclear, but it involves inhibition of phosphodiesterase and an increase in calcium inward flux. The agent also causes some peripheral vasodilation, which may contribute to the cardiac inotropic effect.

155. The answer is D. *(DiPalma, 3/e. p 377. Katzung, 4/e. p 177.)* Lidocaine usually shortens the duration of the action potential and thus allows more time for recovery during diastole. It also blocks both activated and inactivated sodium channels. This has the effect of minimizing the action of lidocaine on normal myocardial tissues as contrasted to depolarized ischemic tissues. Thus lidocaine is particularly suitable for arrhythmias arising during ischemic episodes such as myocardial infarction.

156. The answer is D. *(DiPalma, 3/e. pp 432–433. Katzung, 4/e. p 135.)* Elderly people are apt to have low-reserve kidneys owing to renal artery stenosis. Inhibitors of angiotensin converting enzyme depress renal function and cause proteinuria even in patients with normal kidneys. In the elderly this toxicity is more manifest and may precipitate acute renal failure. The other toxicities listed in the question do not occur at a higher frequency in the elderly.

157. The answer is D. *(DiPalma, 3/e. pp 438–439. Gilman, 8/e. pp 619–620.)* The most likely mechanism of methylxanthine action is by inhibition, not stimulation, of phosphodiesterase. This leads to an increase in cytosolic cyclic AMP and subsequent relaxation of smooth muscle. Methylxanthines also antagonize adenosine receptors. Since adenosine causes bronchoconstriction, this antagonism may also contribute to the bronchodilating action.

158. The answer is D. *(DiPalma, 3/e. p 443. Katzung, 4/e. p 244.)* Cromolyn inhibits the release of mediators from mast cells, including histamine and slow reacting substance of anaphylaxis (SRS-A). This prevents allergically induced bronchospasm. Cromolyn is of no use in an acute asthmatic attack but is of considerable help in prophylaxis of asthmatic attacks, particularly in children.

159. The answer is A. *(DiPalma, 3/e. pp 405–406. Katzung, 4/e. p 428.)* Lovastatin decreases cholesterol synthesis in the liver by inhibiting HMG-CoA reductase, the rate-limiting enzyme in the synthetic pathway. This results in an increase in LDL receptors in the liver, thus reducing blood levels for cholesterol. The intake of dietary cholesterol must not be increased, as this would allow the liver to use more exogenous cholesterol and defeat the action of lovastatin.

160. The answer is B. *(DiPalma, 3/e. p 352. Gilman, 8/e. p 824.)* The usual electrocardiographic pattern of a patient receiving therapeutic doses of digitalis includes an increase in the PR interval, depression and sagging of the ST segment, and occasional biphasia or inversion of the T wave. Symmetrically peaked T waves are associated with hyperkalemia or ischemia in most cases. Shortening of the QT interval, rather than prolongation, is characteristic of digitalis treatment.

161. The answer is B. *(DiPalma, 3/e. p 356. Gilman, 8/e. p 835.)* Low body stores of potassium increase susceptibility to digitalis toxicity. The thiazide diuretics, such as hydrochlorothiazide, promote excretion of potassium. Diuretics are often given with digitoxin to treat congestive heart failure; this combination frequently causes digitalis toxicity.

162. The answer is D. *(DiPalma, 3/e. p 116. Katzung, 4/e. p 834.)* Propranolol as well as other nonselective beta blockers tends to slow the rate of recovery in a hypoglycemic attack caused by insulin. Beta blockers also mask the symptoms of hypoglycemia and may actually cause hypertension because of the increased plasma epinephrine in the presence of vascular $beta_2$ blockade.

163. The answer is D. *(AMA Drug Evaluations Annual 1991, 7/e. pp 535–536. DiPalma, 3/e. pp 385, 390.)* Calcium channel blockers, of which nifedipine is a prime example, are now considered to be more effective than nitrates in relieving variant angina. This is because this type of angina is believed to be caused by vasospasm, which is best antagonized by slow channel calcium blockers. Such blockers appear to have a relative selectivity for coronary arteries.

164. The answer is C. *(DiPalma, 3/e. p 351. Katzung, 4/e. p 155.)* Digitalis inhibits Na^+,K^+-stimulated ATPase and hence decreases the pumping of sodium out of the myocyte. As a result, there is a relative reduction of expulsion of calcium from the cell's sodium-calcium exchange. The consequent increased free calcium in the cell causes increased intensity of interaction between actin and myosin filaments and enhanced contractility.

165. The answer is C. *(DiPalma, 3/e. p 356. Katzung, 4/e. p 159.)* Quinidine is often given in conjunction with digitalis. It has been found by pharmacokinetic studies that this combination results in quinidine's replacing digitalis in tissue binding sites (mainly muscle), thus raising the blood level of digitalis and decreasing its volume of distribution. A mechanism by which quinidine interferes with the renal excretion of digitalis has also been proposed.

166. The answer is A. *(DiPalma, 3/e. p 390. Katzung, 4/e. p 146.)* Verapamil is a prototype drug that acts primarily by interfering with the slow inward movement of calcium into the cardiac muscle cell. It has a significant effect on slow-response characteristics of certain muscle fibers of which the AV nodal tissue is characteristic. Consequently, conduction in AV nodal tissue is depressed while conduction in the Purkinje system is unaffected.

167. The answer is E. *(DiPalma, 3/e. pp 434–435. Katzung, 4/e. p 137.)* Beta blockers are not dilators of peripheral arterioles and lower blood pressure mainly by a negative inotropic effect on the heart. Pindolol, especially, would not be indicated for life-threatening hypertension since it also has $beta_1$-agonist properties. Labetalol is an exception since it has considerable alpha-adrenergic blocking properties in addition to being a beta blocker. Nifedipine is especially useful even by the oral route, as is furosemide, the latter by decreasing blood volume. Diazoxide, although related to thiazide diuretics, does not cause diuresis but is an effective peripheral vasodilator.

168. The answer is B. *(DiPalma, 3/e. pp 260, 273. Katzung, 4/e. p 127.)* Neuronal uptake is necessary for the hypotensive action of guanethidine. It competes for the norepinephrine storage site and in time replaces the natural neurotransmitter. This is the basis of its hypotensive effect. Drugs that prevent reuptake by the neurons, such as cocaine, would destroy the effectiveness of guanethidine.

169. The answer is C. *(DiPalma, 3/e. p 348. Katzung, 4/e. p 219.)* Angiotensin II by a direct mechanism acts on the zona glomerulosa to cause increased conversion of cholesterol to pregnenolone, which results in a greater yield of aldosterone. Angiotensin I is the precursor of angiotensin II. Renin catalyzes the conversion of angiotensin I from angiotensinogen. Kallikreins convert prorenin to active renin. Kininogens are precursors of kinins.

170. The answer is A. *(AMA Drug Evaluations Annual 1991, 7/e. p 635. DiPalma, 3/e. p 471.)* Heparin is a polymer of 8 to 15 sequences of 2 disaccharide units. It is thus a very large molecule, one of the few drugs that does not cross the placenta. Heparin is not secreted in milk and thus is also useful in lactating females. However, heparin's use during pregnancy has not resulted in a lower incidence of maternal hemorrhage or stillbirths as compared with use of coumadin anticoagulants.

171. The answer is B. *(DiPalma, 3/e. pp 123, 418. Katzung, 4/e. p 130.)* Prazosin and its close relative terazosin block mainly alpha$_1$ receptors in contrast to phentolamine, which blocks both alpha$_1$ and alpha$_2$ receptors. The alpha$_1$-receptor selectivity permits the normal norepinephrine negative feedback on alpha$_2$ presynaptic receptors. Pindolol is a beta blocker; minoxidil is a direct-acting vasodilator.

172. The answer is B. *(DiPalma, 3/e. p 422. Katzung, 4/e. p 136.)* Because long-term therapy with diuretics has led to complications of hyperkalemia, uricemia, and hypercholesterolemia, the present approach is to use monotherapy with drugs free of these side effects. Beta blockers (metoprolol), inhibitors of angiotensin converting enzyme (enalapril), and calcium channel blockers (verapamil, nifedipine) are suitable for this purpose. Minoxidil, a direct-acting vasodilator, is indicated in multiple drug therapy in severe hypertension.

173. The answer is B. *(DiPalma, 3/e. p 403. Gilman, 8/e. p 893.)* Nicotinic acid in large doses stimulates the production of prostaglandins as shown by an increase in blood level. The flush may be prevented by the prior administration of aspirin, which is known to block synthesis of prostaglandins.

174. The answer is A. *(DiPalma, 3/e. pp 401–402. Gilman, 8/e. p 881.)* In type I hyperlipoproteinemia, drugs that reduce levels of lipoproteins are not useful, but reduction of dietary sources of fat may help. Cholesterol levels are usually normal but triglycerides are elevated. Maintenance of ideal body weight is recommended in all types of hyperlipidemia. Clofibrate (Atromid-S) effectively reduces the levels of very low-density lipoproteins characteristic of types III, IV, and V hyperlipoproteinemias; and administration of cholestyramine resin and lovastatin in conjunction with a low-cholesterol diet is regarded as effective therapy for type IIa, or primary, hyperbetalipoproteinemia, except in the homozygous familial form.

175. The answer is E. *(DiPalma, 3/e. pp 359, 432–433. Gilman, 8/e. p 758.)* Vasodilator therapy of heart failure has gained prominence in the past 10 years. The angiotensin converting enzyme (ACE) inhibitors (enalapril) are among the best for this purpose, although calcium channel inhibitors and nitroglycerine can also be used. The ACE inhibitors dilate arterioles (reducing preload), dilate veins (reducing preload), and inhibit the production of aldosterone (reduction in blood volume)—all factors considered beneficial in the therapy of congestive heart failure.

176. The answer is C. *(DiPalma, 3/e. pp 371, 376. Gilman, 8/e. p 861.)* Tocainide is chemically a close relative of lidocaine and has the same pharmacologic actions. Drugs classed as IB such as lidocaine, tocainide, and mexiletine are all sodium channel blockers and have local anesthetic activity. They do not appreciably affect refractory period. Tocainide can be given orally in contrast to lidocaine, whose first-pass metabolism limits its use to parenteral therapy.

177. The answer is D. *(DiPalma, 3/e. pp 432–433. Katzung, 4/e. p 135.)* The most consistent of the toxicities of inhibitors of angiotensin converting enzymes is impairment of renal function evidenced by proteinuria. Elevations of BUN and creatinine occur frequently, especially when stenosis of the renal artery or severe heart failure exists. Hyperkalemia also may occur. These drugs are to be used very cautiously where prior renal failure is present and in the elderly. Other toxicities include neutropenia and angioedema. Hepatic toxicity has not been reported.

178. The answer is D. *(DiPalma, 3/e. pp 94, 441, 442. Gilman, 8/e. pp 189, 201.)* Isoproterenol is the most active of the selective beta-sympathomimetic agents. It has virtually no $alpha_1$ or $alpha_2$ activity, yet it manifests potent cardiac inotropic and chronotropic ($beta_1$) as well as vasodilator and bronchodilator ($beta_2$) activity. Usual doses of isoproterenol lower peripheral vascular resistance and diastolic pressure falls; cardiac output is raised, and systolic pressure is generally maintained or increased.

179. The answer is D. *(DiPalma, 3/e. pp 352–353. Gilman, 8/e. pp 824–827.)* Digitalis is used in atrial fibrillation to slow the ventricular rate; the atrial fibrillation itself is not usually controlled. Digitalis acts to slow the speed of conduction and to increase the effective refractory period in the AV node, which prevents transmission of all the impulses from the atria to the ventricles. The drug exerts these effects on the AV node by direct action on the heart and by indirectly increasing vagal activity.

180. The answer is D. *(DiPalma, 3/e. pp 386–387. Gilman, 8/e. pp 765–769.)* Nitroglycerine is the most frequently administered antianginal drug. Its main adverse effects are headache and tachycardia in many patients. By the oral route it undergoes very active first-pass biotransformation and thus is very short-acting. Recently, it has been frequently employed in congestive heart failure because of its property of dilating the venous bed. Despite the fact that nitrates do dilate coronary vessels, most studies show that total coronary flow is not increased (it certainly is not decreased). The sulfhydril group in myocyte membranes converts nitrate to nitrite.

181. The answer is E. *(DiPalma, 3/e. pp 382–383, 391–394. Katzung, 4/e. pp 146, 174, 180.)* Like digitalis, verapamil is most useful in management of supraventricular arrhythmias, including atrial fibrillation, flutter, and atrial tachycardia, especially that caused by reentry mechanisms. It has no clinical use in ventricular arrhythmias. Among its adverse reactions are constipation and headaches, although it also causes bradycardia, hypertension, and cardiac failure. Its main mechanism of action is on the slow-response calcium channels. The oral bioavailability of verapamil is only about 15 percent because of extensive first-pass biotransformation.

182. The answer is B. *(DiPalma, 3/e. p 386. Gilman, 8/e. p 768.)* Adenyl cyclase is not involved. The receptor for nitrite converts NO_2 to NO. This free radical reacts with guanylate cyclase to cause increased synthesis of guanosine 3′-5′-monophosphate (cyclic GMP). A GMP-dependent protein kinase is activated; this results in decreased phosphorylation of muscle protein, which decreases muscle's capacity to contract. In this manner, nitrates relax all smooth muscles. This action of nitrites is identical to that of EDRF.

183. The answer is E. *(DiPalma, 3/e. pp 283, 457, 459, 625. Katzung, 4/e. pp 290, 403, 587, 691.)* Although the cause of pernicious anemia is a deficiency of vitamin B_{12}, deficiency of folic acid may cause a similar syndrome of megaloblastic anemia. In the therapy of cancer, methotrexate—a folate analogue—causes folate deficiency and hence megaloblastic anemia. Trimethoprim is also an antifolate substance used in the chemotherapy of malaria and other bacterial infections. Ordinarily it is quite safe because its affinity for bactericidal folate reductase is greater than for that of the host; however, in large doses it can cause folate deficiency. Phenytoin, a drug widely used to treat epilepsy, can in long-term use bring about folate deficiency possibly by decreasing absorption from the gastrointestinal tract. L-Dopa therapy of Parkinson's disease does not cause megaloblastic anemia.

184. The answer is D. *(DiPalma, 3/e. p 359. Katzung, 4/e. p 132.)* Hydralazine, minoxidil, diazoxide, and sodium nitroprusside are all directly acting vasodilators used to treat hypertension. Because hydralazine, minoxidil, nifedipine, and diazoxide relax arteriolar smooth muscle more than smooth muscle in venules, the effect on venous capacitance is negligible. Sodium nitroprusside, which affects both arterioles and venules, does not increase cardiac output, a feature that enhances the utility of sodium nitroprusside in the management of hypertensive crisis associated with myocardial infarction.

185. The answer is B. *(DiPalma, 3/e. p 375. Gilman, 8/e. pp 856, 857.)* Persons with low hepatic *N*-acetyltransferase activity are known as slow acetylators. A major pathway of metabolism of procainamide, which is used to treat arrhythmias, is *N*-acetylation. Slow acetylators receiving this drug are more susceptible than normal persons to side effects, since slow acetylators will have higher-than-normal blood levels of these drugs. *N*-Acetylprocainamide, the metabolite of procainamide, is also active and is being tested as an antiarrhythmic agent.

186. The answer is C. *(DiPalma, 3/e. pp 97, 366, 371. Gilman, 8/e. pp 195, 818–820.)* Automaticity of Purkinje's fibers is increased by epinephrine, digitalis, isoproterenol, and low concentration of potassium. It is decreased by quinidine or high concentration of potassium. The modification of automaticity is important: in complete heart block, a condition of rhythm failure with bradycardia, isoproterenol or epinephrine might be used to enhance the automaticity of the ventricular conductive system. However, in the situation of supraventricular and ventricular ectopy, all agents able to facilitate automaticity should be avoided.

187. The answer is D. *(DiPalma, 3/e. p 389. Katzung, 4/e. p 148.)* Beta-adrenergic blocking agents do not cause peripheral vasodilation. The lowering of blood pressure is due to a decrease in myocardial contractility. The slowing of heart rate improves the efficiency of the heart, while the buffering effect against sympathetic stimulation prevents sudden increases in oxygen demand. The end result is a heart with a reduced oxygen requirement for a given level of work.

188. The answer is A. *(DiPalma, 3/e. pp 359, 431. Katzung, 4/e. pp 160–161.)* In congestive heart failure the renin-angiotensin-aldosterone system is especially active and it is logical to use inhibitors of angiotensin converting enzyme (captopril, enalapril, lisinopril) to counteract the actions of angiotensin II, which include the stimulation of the adrenals to secrete aldosterone. Inhibitors of angiotensin converting enzyme as vasodilators affect both veins and arteries and thus reduce both preload and afterload. They do not result in development of tolerance as do the nitrates. One disadvantage is that they do cause renal toxicity, and this limits their use to patients with good renal function.

189. The answer is D. *(DiPalma, 3/e. pp 453–454. Katzung, 4/e. pp 396–397.)* Iron deficiency anemia usually occurs in infants undergoing rapid growth. In adults in a late stage it may result in a bowel syndrome associated with gastritis and hypochlorhydria (Plummer-Vinson syndrome). Characteristically all iron deficiency anemias are associated with a hypochromic microcytic blood profile. Infestation with the tapeworm *Diphyllobothrium latum* is accompanied by a hyperchromic macrocytic anemia treatable with vitamin B_{12}. Bleeding syndromes are treated with iron.

190. The answer is D. *(DiPalma, 3/e. p 357. Gilman, 8/e. pp 835–836.)* In digitalis overdose only the administration of a specific Fab fragment that acts as an antibody for digitalis is effective. This raises the blood level of the digitalis glycoside but it is not available for action on the heart and indeed the combined Fab fragment–digitalis complex is excreted by the kidney. While potassium, magnesium, and phenytoin will counteract some of the arrhythmogenic actions of digitalis, they are not effective in severe digitalis overdose. Calcium would augment the toxicity of digitalis.

191. The answer is E. *(DiPalma, 3/e. pp 386–387. Katzung, 4/e. p 143.)* There is no doubt that, experimentally, nitrates dilate coronary vessels. This also occurs in normal subjects, resulting in an overall increase in coronary blood flow. In arteriosclerotic coronaries, the ability to dilate is lost and the ischemic area may actually have less blood flow under the influence of nitrates. Improvement in the ischemic condition is the result of decreased myocardial oxygen demands because of a reduction of preload and afterload. Nitrates dilate both arteries and veins and thus reduce the work of the heart. As the blood pressure falls, there is reflex tachycardia. Nitrates are compatible with beta blockers, which slow the heart and counteract the reflex tachycardia caused by nitrates.

192. The answer is B. *(DiPalma, 3/e. pp 355–356. Katzung, 4/e. pp 146–147. Wilson, 12/e. p 1225.)* Smooth muscle, especially of vasculature, depends on transmembrane calcium influx for normal resting tone and contractile responses. In contrast, skeletal muscle uses intracellular pools of calcium and does not depend on calcium influx. Cardiac muscle requires calcium influx for excitation-contraction coupling. A reduction in mechanical function of the myocardium reduces the oxygen requirement in angina pectoris. Calcium influx is required for the release of several hormones, for example insulin. However, the doses required are too large to be used routinely in humans. Esophageal spasm may be combated by nifedipine.

193. The answer is D. *(DiPalma, 3/e. pp 469, 477–479. Gilman, 8/e. p 1323. Katzung, 4/e. p 412.)* Tissue plasminogen activator, urokinase, and streptokinase, although obtained from different sources, all are capable of dissolving a fibrin clot. Tissue plasminogen activator is manufactured by a recombinant technique and is extremely expensive. It may have the advantage of causing less cerebral bleeding as compared with streptokinase and urokinase. Factor IX complex is a dried human plasma fraction that is used to promote clotting when a bleeding episode caused by a genetic acquired deficiency of these factors is evident. A combination of streptokinase and lys-plasminogen, anistreplase, has been recently introduced and may have advantages over tissue plasminogen activator or streptokinase used alone.

194. The answer is C. *(DiPalma, 3/e. pp 454, 458–462. Gilman, 8/e. pp 1294–1306.)* Vitamin B_{12} deficiency has several causes. Pernicious anemia, associated with gastric mucosal atrophy and histamine-refractory achlorhydria, eliminates the production of intrinsic factor that would combine with cyanocobalamin (B_{12}) in the gut. Parenteral administration of B_{12} is recommended for patients who have pernicious anemia. Oral B_{12} and intrinsic factor concentrate should be used only in patients who have a proven intrinsic factor deficit and refuse intramuscular administration of B_{12}. Other causes of vitamin B_{12} deficiency, in the face of normal intrinsic factor secretion, include malabsorption syndromes and parasitic competition. Alcohol-associated megaloblastic anemia is usually caused by a deficiency of folic acid. Folinic acid is used to circumvent the effects of inhibitors of dehydrofolate reductase such as methotrexate.

195. The answer is E. *(DiPalma, 3/e. pp 471–472. Gilman, 8/e. p 1313.)* Heparin, a naturally occurring anticoagulant, is localized largely in mast cells.

A mucopolysaccharide, it is composed of sulfated glucosamine and glucuronic acid. Its primary action is as an antithrombin factor, for which it requires a plasma cofactor. Organic bases (protamine) are believed to inhibit heparin by neutralizing its electronegative charge. Heparin is thought to release and stabilize a lipemia-clearing factor that catalyzes the hydrolysis of triglycerides. It does not cross the placental barrier and thus can be used as an anticoagulant during pregnancy.

196. The answer is A. *(DiPalma, 3/e. pp 406–407. Katzung, 4/e. p 428.)* Lovastatin should not be used in patients with severe liver disease. With routine use of lovastatin, serum transaminase values may rise, and in such patients the drug may be continued only with great caution. Lovastatin has also been associated with lenticular opacities, and slit-lamp studies should be done before and 1 year after the start of therapy. There is no effect on the otic nerve. The drug is not toxic to the renal system and reports of bone marrow depression are very rare. There is a small incidence of myopathy, and levels of creatinine kinase should be measured when unexplained muscle pain occurs. Combination with cyclosporine or clofibrate has led to myopathy. There is no danger in use with bile acid sequestrants.

197. The answer is A. *(DiPalma, 3/e. p 383. Katzung, 4/e. p 180.)* Verapamil has replaced all other older forms of therapy for supraventricular tachycardias. Older therapies—all designed to favor parasympathetic control of rhythm—include digitalis, propranolol, edrophonium, and vasoconstrictors. The vasoconstrictor phenylephrine (given by intravenous bolus) causes stimulation of the carotid sinus and reflex vagal stimulation of the atria. More recently, adenosine has been favored over verapamil.

198. The answer is B. *(DiPalma, 3/e. pp 390–391. Katzung, 4/e. pp 147–148.)* The available agents for blocking calcium influx include verapamil, nifedipine, and diltiazem. Among these drugs, nifedipine has the least effect on atrioventricular conduction and therefore is preferred in the presence of conduction abnormalities in this location. All the blockers of calcium influx are capable of negative inotropic effects on cardiac contractility at high dosage. At doses that cause arteriolar dilatation, myocardial contractility is not affected. Thus, these agents can be used in the presence of heart failure. Verapamil has distinct antiarrhythmic properties, especially in supraventricular arrhythmias. Nifedipine causes the most arteriolar dilatation and as a consequence is contraindicated in patients with low blood pressure. Paradoxically nifedipine may be the best choice in patients with depressed left ventricular function, as it reduces afterload by reducing arteriolar resistance. Use of calcium channel blockers with beta-adrenergic blockers causes excessive cardiac depression.

199–202. The answers are: 199-C, 200-A, 201-B, 202-D. *(DiPalma, 3/e. pp 402–407. Gilman, 8/e. pp 881–894.)* Cholestyramine is an anion-exchange resin that is not absorbed. It binds bile acids in the intestine and increases fecal excretion of the acids. Cholestyramine must be combined with a low-cholesterol diet to be effective.

Gemfibrozil is chemically related to clofibrate and apparently works in a similar fashion. Like clofibrate it lowers the level of very low-density lipoproteins (VLDLs) in the plasma, but unlike clofibrate it elevates high-density lipoproteins (HDLs). The agent inhibits lipolysis of stored triglyceride in adipose tissue.

Lovastatin has the most specific mechanism of action as it is an effective inhibitor of HMB-CoA reductase at a rate-limiting step in cholesterol synthesis. Low-density lipoproteins (LDLs) are decreased and HDLs are increased in the blood.

Nicotinic acid is an older drug that decreases the production of VLDL in the liver and lowers the blood level of LDL. The total synthesis of cholesterol in the body is not decreased and nicotinic acid therapy is best combined with other cholesterol-reducing drugs and a low-cholesterol diet. Nicotinic acid does not significantly alter excretion of bile acids. While nicotinic acid does inhibit lipolysis, it also decreases esterification of triglycerides in the liver.

203–207. The answers are: 203-C, 204-A, 205-E, 206-F, 207-B. *(DiPalma, 3/e. pp 98, 105, 359, 389, 443. Gilman, 8/e. pp 161, 173, 798, 813, 1483.)* Isoproterenol, a catecholamine that acts on beta-adrenergic receptors, is given parenterally because absorption after sublingual or oral administration is unreliable. It is a synthetic sympathomimetic structurally similar to epinephrine. Isoproterenol produces myocardial stimulation and is used for the treatment of atrioventricular heart block, cardiogenic shock associated with myocardial infarction, cardiac arrest, and septicemic shock.

Terbutaline is a synthetic sympathomimetic amine that acts on the beta-adrenergic receptors of bronchial smooth muscle and causes a decrease in airway and pulmonary resistance. Oral doses are effective for management of bronchial asthma and for the reversible bronchospasm that may occur in bronchitis and emphysema. Terbutaline has a modest therapeutic advantage over a less selective bronchodilator.

The coronary vasodilator nitroglycerine may be administered orally, sublingually, topically, intravenously, and most recently transdermally. Its small dose and molecular structure permit its passage through the skin. This is accomplished by attaching a nitroglycerine-containing, multilayered film to the skin.

Beclomethasone is a glucocorticoid especially designed for aerosol administration. This permits its therapeutic action in the lungs while minimizing systemic effects. Great care must be exercised when transferring patients from systemic corticosteroids to beclomethasone because fatal adrenal insufficiency has occurred in asthmatic patients undergoing such transfer.

Sodium nitroprusside can only be administered intravenously. It is an effective vasodilator for heart failure because it dilates both arterioles and veins and thus reduces both preload and afterload. Maximal onset of action is in 1 to 2 min, and the effect dissipates rapidly when infusion is stopped.

Cromolyn sodium is inhaled as a powder administered by a special device ("turbo-inhaler").

208–212. The answers are: 208-G, 209-B, 210-F, 211-H, 212-C. *(DiPalma, 3/e. pp 362, 371. Katzung, 4/e. pp 173–174.)* It is widely accepted that antiarrhythmic drugs are best classified according to their electrophysiologic attributes. This is best accomplished by relating the effects of the different drugs to their actions on sodium and calcium channels, which are reflected by changes in the monophasic action potential.

Amiodarone blocks sodium channels and markedly prolongs repolarization, particularly in depolarized cells. Flecainide is related to local anesthetics and also affects sodium channels, but has little effect on repolarization. Mexiletine, which is in the same group of local anesthetics as lidocaine, is remarkable because it either does not affect or shortens repolarization. Its action is mainly on depolarized fibers. Disopyramide slows depolarization and repolarization and, like quinidine, delays conduction. Verapamil, a calcium channel blocker, affects the resting potential or phase 4 and thus has its greatest effect on pacemaker tissue; it is mainly of utility in supraventricular arrhythmias. Digitalis also affects phase 4 of the action potential, but it also greatly hastens repolarization. Although nifedipine is a calcium channel blocker, it has little effect on the electrophysiology of the heart. Propranolol has actions mainly on slow response fibers and suppresses automaticity.

213–217. The answers are: 213-C, 214-D, 215-F, 216-B, 217-E. *(DiPalma, 3/e. pp 395, 471–474, 476–478, 495, 692. Gilman, 8/e. pp 1314–1316, 1317–1322, 1323–1327.)* Heparin's action as an antithrombin factor requires the presence of an $alpha_2$ globulin, antithrombin III. Antithrombin III is a protease inhibitor that inhibits the activity of several of the clotting factors by forming irreversible complexes. Heparin facilitates the formation of these complexes and is antagonized by protamine sulfate.

Coumarin derivatives antagonize vitamin K and cause a decrease in production of prothrombin and coagulation factors VII, IX, and X. Oral anticoagulants prevent formation of these factors by blocking formation of the reduced form of vitamin K.

Dipyridamole is classified as a coronary vasodilator. Its effectiveness in inhibiting platelet aggregation and adhesion has been proved in vitro but has still to be demonstrated in vivo. Dipyridamole is used in patients with prosthetic heart valves as primary prophylaxis against thromboemboli. It is used in combination with warfarin.

Streptokinase is obtained from group-C β-hemolytic streptococci. Both urokinase and streptokinase activate plasminogen to plasmin, which is a protease. Plasmin dissolves thrombin by breaking down fibrin.

Ethylenediaminetetraacetic acid (EDTA) inactivates calcium in vitro by forming a complex with the calcium, thus preventing clotting. This approach is impossible in vivo because calcium levels that are low enough to prevent coagulation also are low enough to be lethal.

Factor IX complex is a procoagulant drug mainly used in patients with hemophilia B.

218–222. The answers are: 218-B, 219-D, 220-E, 221-A, 222-B. *(DiPalma, 3/e. pp 423, 430–432. Gilman, 8/e. pp 208–209, 749–752.)* The enzyme renin acts upon angiotensinogen (an alpha globulin) to yield the decapeptide angiotensin I, which has limited pharmacologic activity. Angiotensin I is metabolized extensively in a single passage through the lungs by the carboxypeptidase peptidyl dipeptidase (also called *kinase II*, or *angiotensin converting enzyme*) to the octapeptide angiotensin II.

Angiotensin II has a potent direct action on the vascular smooth muscle and also indirectly stimulates contraction by means of the sympathetic nervous system. The vasoconstriction in response to angiotensin II involves precapillary arterioles and postcapillary venules and results in an increased total peripheral resistance.

The octapeptide saralasin is an analogue of angiotensin II and has an alanine in place of the phenylalanine in the 8 position. It is a potent antagonist of angiotensin II and, thus, can reduce elevated blood pressure in patients with significant amounts of circulating angiotensin II (i.e., renin-dependent hypertension). Being a polypeptide, saralasin must be administered intravenously, which limits its therapeutic use.

Captopril and clonidine, in contrast, are orally effective antihypertensive agents. Captopril (D-3-mercapto-methylpropanoyl-L-proline) is a rationally designed, competitive inhibitor of peptidyl dipeptidase. Unlike saralasin, it blocks the formation but not the response of angiotensin II. Captopril is useful in reducing the blood pressure of both renin-dependent and normal-renin essential hypertension. The hypotensive action of clonidine is believed to be due primarily to stimulation of the alpha-adrenergic receptors in the central nervous system (CNS). A reduction in the discharge rate of preganglionic adrenergic nerves occurs in addition to bradycardia. The CNS actions of clonidine also lead to a reduction in the level of renin activity in the plasma.

Central Nervous System

- General Anesthetics
  - Halothane
  - Euflurane
  - Isoflurane
  - Methoxyflurane
  - Nitrous oxide
- Intravenous Anesthetics
  - Thiopental
  - Methohexital
  - Midazolam
  - Ketamine
  - Etomidate
  - Fentanyl
- Sedatives and Hypnotics
  - Barbiturates
    - Amobarbital
    - Butabarbital
    - Secobarbital
    - Mephobarbital
    - Metharbital
    - Phenobarbital
  - Benzodiazepines
    - Flurazepam
    - Temazepam
    - Triazolam
  - Miscellaneous group
    - Chloral hydrate
    - Paraldehyde
    - Ethchlorvynol
    - Ethinamate
    - Glutethimide
- Antianxiety Drugs
  - Benzodiazepines
    - Chlordiazepoxide*
    - Diazepam*
    - Clorazepate
    - Halazepam
    - Lorazepam
    - Oxazepam
    - Prazepam
    - Alprazolam
  - Propanediols
    - Meprobamate
  - Miscellaneous
    - Buspirone
    - Hydroxyzine
- Ethanol and Related Alcohols
  - Ethanol
  - Ethylene glycol
  - Isopropyl alcohol
  - Methanol
  - Disulfiram as a deterrent
- Psychotomimetic Drugs
  - Lysergic acid diethylamide (LSD)
  - Mescaline
  - Psilocybin
  - Phencyclidine
  - Amphetamine
  - Methamphetamine
  - Cocaine
  - Marijuana
- Antipsychotic Drugs
  - Phenothiazines
    - Promazine
    - Chlorpromazine*
    - Triflupromazine
    - Prochlorperazine
    - Trifluoperazine
    - Fluphenazine
    - Thioridazine
  - Thioxanthene derivatives
    - Chlorprothixene
    - Thiothixene
  - Butyrophenone
    - Haloperidol
    - Miscellaneous group
    - Molindone
    - Loxapine

- Pimozide
- Lithium carbonate

Antidepressant Drugs

- Tricyclics
  - Imipramine*
  - Amitriptyline
  - Desipramine
  - Nortriptyline
  - Protriptyline
  - Trimipramine
  - Doxepin
- Monoamine oxidase inhibitors
  - Tranylcypromine
  - Phenelzine
  - Isocarboxazid
- Second-generation antidepressants
  - Maprotiline
  - Amoxapine
  - Trazodone
  - Fluoxetine

Antiepileptic and Antiparkinsonism Drugs

- Tonic-clonic and focal seizures
  - Phenytoin,* mephenytoin
  - Carbamazepine
  - Phenobarbital
  - Primidone
- Absence seizures
  - Ethosuximide*
  - Valproic acid*
  - Clonazepam
  - Acetazolamide
  - Trimethadione
- Anticholinergics for parkinsonism
  - Trihexyphenidyl*
  - Procyclidine
  - Biperiden
  - Benztropine*
  - Diphenhydramine
  - Orphenadrine
- Levodopa for parkinsonism
  - Selegiline*
- Miscellaneous agents for parkinsonism
  - Amantadine
  - Bromocriptine

Narcotic Analgesics

- Endogenous opioid peptides
  - Met- and leu-enkephalin
  - β-Endorphin
  - Dynorphin
- Agonists
  - Morphine*
  - Codeine*
  - Heroin
  - Hydromorphone
  - Oxymorphone
  - Oxycodone
  - Levorphanol
  - Meperidine, methadone
  - Propoxyphene
- Antagonists
  - Naloxone
  - Naltrexone
- Mixed agonists-antagonists
  - Buprenorphine
  - Butorphanol
  - Nalbuphine
  - Pentazocine

Nonnarcotic Analgesics

- Salicylates
- Aspirin
- Diflunisal
- Magnesium salicylate
- Salsalate
- Propionic acids
  - Fenoprofen
  - Ibuprofen
  - Ketoprofen
  - Naproxen
- Acetic acids
  - Indomethacin
  - Sulindac
  - Tolmetin
  - Diclofenac
- Oxicams
  - Piroxicam
- Pyrazolone
  - Phenylbutazone
- Fenamates
  - Meclofenamate
  - Mefenamic acid

Local Anesthetics
- Esters
  - Cocaine
  - Procaine
  - Chloroprocaine
  - Tetracaine
- Amides
  - Lidocaine*
  - Mepivacaine
  - Bupivacaine
  - Etidocaine
  - Prilocaine

Drug Dependence
- Terms
  - Psychological dependence
  - Addiction
  - Physical dependence
  - Drug abuse
  - Tolerance

Schedules of Drug Enforcement Administration
- Numbers I to VI

Stimulants
- Cocaine and amphetamines
- Hallucinogens (LSD)
- Marijuana

DIRECTIONS: Each question below contains five suggested responses. Select the **one best** response to each question.

223. All the following compounds are indicated for the treatment of psychoses EXCEPT

(A) perphenazine (Trilafon)
(B) thiothixene hydrochloride (Navane)
(C) fluoxetine hydrochloride (Prozac)
(D) haloperidol (Haldol)
(E) loxapine succinate (Loxitane)

224. The use of morphine is contraindicated in

(A) myocardial infarction
(B) cor pulmonale
(C) dysentery
(D) migraine headache
(E) acute pulmonary edema

225. All the following statements are true about triazolam EXCEPT

(A) it binds to benzodiazepine receptor, enhancing GABA-mediated chloride influx
(B) it is useful in the treatment of insomnia
(C) it enhances the activity of the drug-metabolizing microsomal system
(D) combined with ethanol, it may produce significant respiratory depression
(E) adverse effects may include drowsiness, dizziness, lethargy, and ataxia

226. All the following statements are true concerning phenelzine sulfate (Nardil) EXCEPT that the drug

(A) has antidepressant properties
(B) can produce orthostatic hypotension
(C) irreversibly inhibits monamine oxidases
(D) can induce hypertensive crises when aged cheese, beer, or pickled herring is ingested
(E) has prominent adverse effects including dry mouth, constipation, blurred vision, and urinary retention

227. Which of the following local anesthetics is useful for topical (surface) administration *only*?

(A) Procaine
(B) Bupivacaine
(C) Etidocaine
(D) Benzocaine
(E) Lidocaine

228. Akathisia, Parkinson-like syndrome, galactorrhea, and amenorrhea are side effects of perphenazine caused by

(A) blockade of muscarinic receptors
(B) blockade of alpha-adrenergic receptors
(C) blockade of dopamine receptors
(D) supersensitivity of dopamine receptors
(E) stimulation of nicotinic receptors

229. All the following statements are true about mepivacaine EXCEPT

(A) it acts by interfering with sodium influx in nerve fibers
(B) coadministration of epinephrine would prolong its duration of action
(C) adverse reactions to its use may include CNS and cardiovascular depression
(D) it is biotransformed by plasma esterases
(E) it is slowly metabolized in the fetus and neonate

230. Which of the following agents is useful in treatment of malignant hyperthermia?

(A) Baclofen
(B) Diazepam
(C) Cyclobenzaprine
(D) Dantrolene
(E) Halothane

231. The agent most effective in acute treatment of migraine headache is

(A) propranolol
(B) methysergide
(C) clonidine
(D) ergotamine tartrate
(E) amitriptyline

232. Which of the following is an antidepressant agent that selectively inhibits serotonin (5-HT) uptake with minimal effect on norepinephrine uptake?

(A) Protriptyline
(B) Maprotiline
(C) Fluoxetine
(D) Desipramine
(E) Amoxapine

233. All the following benzodiazepines are biotransformed to active products EXCEPT

(A) alprazolam
(B) diazepam
(C) oxazepam
(D) prazepam
(E) chlordiazepoxide

234. Effects of thioridazine include all the following EXCEPT

(A) orthostatic hypotension, constipation, and urinary retention
(B) tardive dyskinesia
(C) hypoprolactinemia
(D) antiemesis
(E) control of psychotic behavior

235. All the following statements about chloral hydrate are true EXCEPT that it

(A) irritates the gastric mucosa
(B) produces physical dependence
(C) produces hypnosis rapidly
(D) effectively produces analgesia
(E) accelerates the biotransformation of some drugs by the hepatic microsomal metabolizing system

236. A high degree of tolerance develops to all the following effects of hydromorphone EXCEPT

(A) euphoria
(B) analgesia
(C) nausea and vomiting
(D) respiratory depression
(E) constipation

237. Which of the following inhalation anesthetics is most likely to produce diffusion hypoxia?

(A) Isoflurane
(B) Enflurane
(C) Methoxyflurane
(D) Halothane
(E) Nitrous oxide

238. Carbidopa is useful in the treatment of Parkinson's disease because it

(A) is a precursor of L-dopa
(B) is a dopaminergic receptor agonist
(C) prevents peripheral biotransformation of L-dopa
(D) prevents breakdown of dopamine
(E) promotes a decreased concentration of L-dopa in the nigrostriatum

239. Ketamine produces all the following effects EXCEPT

(A) profound analgesia
(B) amnesia
(C) mild increase in muscle tone
(D) disorientation, illusions, and vivid dreams on emergence
(E) cardiovascular depression

240. Which of the following drugs mimics the activity of met-enkephalin in the dorsal horn of the spinal cord?

(A) Selegiline
(B) Trihexyphenidyl
(C) Baclofen
(D) Morphine
(E) Phenobarbital

241. The preferred treatment of status epilepticus is intravenous administration of

(A) chlorpromazine
(B) diazepam
(C) succinylcholine
(D) tranylcypromine
(E) ethosuximide

242. All the following statements about methadone are true EXCEPT

(A) it is useful as an analgesic
(B) it has greater oral efficacy than morphine
(C) it possesses opioid antagonist effects
(D) it produces a milder but more protracted withdrawal syndrome than that associated with morphine
(E) adverse reactions may include constipation, respiratory depression, and lightheadedness

243. All the following statements are true about amphetamine EXCEPT that it

(A) releases catecholamines from central and peripheral adrenergic neurons
(B) may cause tachycardia, cardiac arrhythmias, and anginal pain
(C) is used in the treatment of narcolepsy
(D) is rapidly biotransformed by catechol-*O*-methyltransferase (COMT)
(E) can lead to toxic psychosis, hyperthermia, and hypertension

244. The effect of tranylcypromine can be attributed to

(A) a direct nicotinelike stimulation
(B) inhibition of serotonin uptake
(C) a xanthinelike stimulation
(D) the inhibition of monoamine oxidase
(E) blockade of dopamine receptors

245. Desipramine can produce all the following EXCEPT

(A) sedation
(B) xerostomia and constipation
(C) anticonvulsant effect
(D) orthostatic hypotension
(E) decrease in REM sleep

246. All the following statements are true about thiopental EXCEPT that it

(A) is ultra-short-acting by virtue of redistribution
(B) sensitizes the myocardium to endogenous catecholamines
(C) may cause laryngospasm and bronchospasm
(D) is biotransformed to pentobarbital
(E) produces little postanesthetic excitement or vomiting

247. All the following statements are true about ethanol EXCEPT

(A) it is a hepatotoxic agent
(B) it elevates body temperature by peripheral vasoconstriction
(C) it suppresses the release of antidiuretic hormone
(D) it can lead to gastritis and pancreatitis
(E) acute overdose can cause acidosis, hypoglycemia, and elevated intracranial pressure

248. Which of the following statements correctly characterizes buspirone?

(A) It enhances the affinity of GABA for its receptor
(B) It has potent anticonvulsant properties
(C) It possesses skeletal muscle relaxant properties
(D) It is useful in management of anxiety states
(E) It produces a parkinsonian syndrome

249. Which of the following is a selective inhibitor of monoamine oxidase B useful in the treatment of parkinsonism?

(A) Bromocriptine
(B) Carbidopa
(C) Deprenyl (selegiline)
(D) Phenelzine
(E) Tranylcypromine

250. All the following statements are true concerning bupropion hydrochloride (Wellbutrin) EXCEPT that the drug

(A) is indicated for the treatment of depression
(B) is a potent inhibitor of both norepinephrine and serotonin reuptake into noradrenergic and serotonergic neurons, respectively
(C) has no significant anticholinergic activity
(D) produces stimulant effects on the central nervous system (CNS) that may result in seizures at elevated dosage regimens
(E) is biotransformed to several products, two of which are pharmacologically active

251. All the following statements about lidocaine (Xylocaine) are true EXCEPT

(A) it is biotransformed by amidase
(B) vasodilation increases duration of action
(C) it has rapid onset of action
(D) topical application can produce surface anesthesia
(E) it can be used to induce epidural anesthesia

252. All the following statements are true of clorazepate EXCEPT that it

(A) may cause psychological dependence
(B) is activated in the stomach
(C) is useful as an antianxiety agent
(D) has a duration of action of less than 10 h
(E) is chemically a benzodiazepine

253. Which of the following statements is true concerning abuse of opioid analgesics?

(A) No cross tolerance develops among opioid analgesics
(B) Tolerance develops equally to all effects of opioids
(C) Opioids reduce pain, aggression, and sexual drives
(D) The symptoms of acute methadone withdrawal are qualitatively different from those of acute heroin withdrawal
(E) None of the above

254. All the following statements are true of benzodiazepine derivatives EXCEPT

(A) flurazepam is useful for insomnia
(B) diazepam is useful for symptoms of acute alcohol withdrawal
(C) lorazepam is useful as a premedication for endoscopy
(D) clonazepam is useful for generalized tonic-clonic seizures
(E) chlordiazepoxide is useful as a long-acting antianxiety agent

255. Neuroleptic malignant syndrome is associated with use of

(A) oxazepam (Serax)
(B) amobarbital (Amytal)
(C) doxepin hydrochloride (Sinequan)
(D) trifluoperazine hydrochloride (Stelazine)
(E) phenytoin (Dilantin)

256. A drug that specifically enhances metabolically the activity of brain dopamine is

(A) benztropine
(B) selegiline
(C) trihexyphenidyl
(D) bromocriptine
(E) chlorpromazine

257. The pharmacologic properties of acetylsalicylic acid include

(A) a rapid and effective reduction in elevated temperature
(B) promotion of platelet aggregation
(C) alleviation of pain by stimulation of prostaglandin synthesis
(D) potency equal to that of acetaminophen as an anti-inflammatory agent
(E) less gastric irritation than other salicylates

258. In addition to its use in the treatment of schizophrenia, chlorpromazine (Thorazine) is effective

(A) in reducing nausea and vomiting
(B) as an antihypertensive agent
(C) as an antihistaminic
(D) in the treatment of depression
(E) for treating bipolar affective disorder

259. All the following are true concerning maprotiline hydrochloride (Ludiomil) EXCEPT that it

(A) has antidepressant effects
(B) selectively blocks norepinephrine reuptake into presynaptic nerve terminals
(C) may cause constipation, blurred vision, and tachycardia
(D) may induce sedation
(E) inhibits monoamine oxidase

260. Nalbuphine may be characterized by which of the following statements?

(A) It has analgesic properties equipotent to morphine
(B) It inhibits withdrawal symptoms in persons dependent on morphine
(C) At high doses, respiratory depression with nalbuphine is equal to that seen with morphine
(D) It is a pure opioid antagonist at μ, κ, and σ receptors
(E) It has an addiction potential equal to morphine

261. All the following are characteristics of lithium carbonate EXCEPT that it

(A) has a general sedation action similar to that of the phenothiazine derivatives
(B) may induce tremors and nephrogenic diabetes insipidus
(C) is useful in the treatment of bipolar affective (manic-depressive) disorders
(D) has a low therapeutic index, and plasma or serum concentrations must be determined to facilitate safe use of the drug
(E) will accumulate in patients who are taking any diuretic that will cause significant Na^+ depletion

262. Cocaine, produced from the leaves of *Erythroxylon* species,

(A) produces bradycardia and vasodilation
(B) is directly related chemically to opioid analgesics
(C) is metabolized by the microsomal metabolizing system
(D) effectively blocks nerve conduction
(E) blocks norepinephrine receptors directly

263. A drug of choice for the therapy of absence seizures is

(A) phenobarbital
(B) phenytoin
(C) carbamazepine
(D) ethosuximide
(E) trimethadione

264. Which of the following agents is a selective D_2 (dopamine receptor) agonist?

(A) Fluphenazine
(B) Bromocriptine
(C) Promethazine
(D) Haloperidol
(E) Chlorpromazine

265. A patient is diagnosed as having Tourette's syndrome. The drug of choice for the treatment of this disease is

(A) chlorpromazine hydrochloride (Thorazine)
(B) fluphenazine hydrochloride (Prolixin)
(C) haloperidol (Haldol)
(D) pimozide (Orap)
(E) chlorprothixene (Taractan)

266. All the following agents enhance the activity of γ-aminobutyric acid (GABA) EXCEPT

(A) chlordiazepoxide
(B) phenobarbital
(C) halazepam
(D) valproic acid
(E) chlorpromazine

267. All the following statements regarding marijuana are true EXCEPT

(A) it may lower intraocular pressure
(B) a sign of acute intoxication is reddening of conjunctiva
(C) it has antiemetic properties
(D) heavy chronic use can lower serum testosterone levels in men
(E) it causes flashbacks

268. All the following drugs produce an abstinence syndrome characterized as being excitatory EXCEPT

(A) morphine
(B) ethanol
(C) phenobarbital
(D) cocaine
(E) glutethimide

269. Naltrexone, a widely used agent in the rehabilitation of opioid-dependent patients, has all the following characteristics EXCEPT

(A) it lacks opioid agonist activity at therapeutic doses
(B) it possesses longer duration of action than naloxone
(C) it will precipitate withdrawal syndrome in a heroin addict
(D) it is usually administered intravenously
(E) it is subject to "first-pass" metabolism in the liver

270. Drugs that produce their pharmacologic effects by inhibition of prostaglandin synthesis include all the following EXCEPT

(A) indomethacin
(B) ibuprofen
(C) acetaminophen
(D) piroxicam
(E) naproxen

271. All the following are a consequence of ethanol abuse EXCEPT

(A) development of metabolic tolerance
(B) reduced effect of barbiturates in an intoxicated alcoholic person
(C) possible development of disorientation, tremors, hallucinations, and convulsions when consumption of ethanol is abruptly ended
(D) hepatitis
(E) pancreatitis

272. All the following statements regarding barbiturates are true EXCEPT

(A) pentobarbital is a biotransformation product of thiopental
(B) phenobarbital can decrease the enzymatic activity of δ-aminolevulinic acid
(C) mephobarbital can be used in the treatment of tonic-clonic seizures
(D) the duration of effect for methohexital is determined by redistribution
(E) alkalinization of the urine readily enhances the excretion of secobarbital

273. Correct statements concerning fentanyl include all the following EXCEPT

(A) it has been shown to be up to 100 times more potent than morphine
(B) it is usually administered orally
(C) it is useful for anesthesia
(D) at high doses it produces muscular rigidity, which is reversed by naloxone
(E) it is combined with droperidol to produce neuroleptanalgesia

274. All the following statements are true of halothane (Fluothane) EXCEPT that it

(A) is more potent as an anesthetic than nitrous oxide
(B) increases cardiac output
(C) causes respiratory depression with increased anesthetic levels
(D) may produce hepatotoxicity
(E) is a halogenated alkane

275. True statements about mechanisms of drugs used in the treatment of parkinsonism include all the following EXCEPT

(A) benztropine blocks muscarinic receptors
(B) amantadine stimulates release of dopamine from storage sites
(C) bromocriptine stimulates dopaminergic receptors
(D) levodopa enhances the synthesis of dopamine
(E) selegiline is an inhibitor of monoamine oxidase A

276. True statements about codeine include all the following EXCEPT that it

(A) produces naloxone-reversible respiratory depression
(B) may cause hypotension as a result of histamine release
(C) has antitussive properties
(D) is exempt from the narcotics control laws
(E) is partially biotransformed to morphine

277. True statements regarding naloxone include all the following EXCEPT

(A) it reverses the analgesic effects of butorphanol
(B) it is useful for the treatment of opiate overdose
(C) it induces withdrawal symptoms in a heroin addict
(D) it reverses phenobarbital-induced respiratory depression
(E) it has poor oral bioavailability

278. A correct statement regarding alprazolam is that it

(A) potentiates the activity of dopamine as its major mechanism of action
(B) is more potent than diazepam in relieving skeletal muscle spasm
(C) is useful in the management of anxiety
(D) causes more severe respiratory depression than does phenobarbital
(E) is classified as a long-acting phenothiazine derivative

279. Which of the following statements about "crack" (the free-base form of cocaine) is true?

(A) "Flashbacks" (recurrences of effects) may occur months after the last use of the drug
(B) It may cause seizures and cardiac arrhythmias
(C) It acts by blocking adrenergic receptors
(D) It is the salt form of cocaine
(E) It is primarily administered intranasally

280. Treatment of phencyclidine overdose may include administration of

(A) amitriptyline
(B) haloperidol
(C) physostigmine
(D) sodium bicarbonate
(E) amphetamine

DIRECTIONS: Each group of questions below consists of lettered headings followed by a set of numbered items. For each numbered item select the **one** lettered heading with which it is **most** closely associated. Each lettered heading may be used **once, more than once, or not at all.**

Questions 281–283

Match each description with the appropriate drug.

(A) Isocarboxazid (Marplan)
(B) Trazodone (Desyrel)
(C) Mesoridazine (Serentil)
(D) Pimozide (Orap)
(E) Amitriptyline (Elavil)
(F) Fluoxetine (Prozac)
(G) Protriptyline (Vivactil)
(H) Amoxapine (Asendin)
(I) Clozapine (Clozaril)
(J) Nortriptyline (Aventyl)
(K) Fluphenazine (Prolixin)
(L) Molindone (Moban)

281. This tricyclic antidepressant has high anticholinergic activity, is one of the more sedating compounds of the group, and is biotransformed to a long-acting active product

282. Relatively insoluble salts of this antipsychotic drug have been prepared for use as intramuscular depot injections

283. This drug has the lowest incidence of extrapyramidal reactions, but the highest incidence of agranulocytosis, of all the antipsychotic compounds

Questions 284–286

Match each description with the appropriate drug.

(A) Primidone
(B) Disulfiram
(C) Dextroamphetamine
(D) Valproic acid
(E) Flurazepam
(F) Phenylephrine
(G) Phenytoin
(H) Isoetharine
(I) Carbamazepine
(J) Amitriptyline
(K) Triazolam
(L) Diazepam

284. Causes megaloblastic anemia, ataxia, and gingival hyperplasia

285. Is used in the management of ethanol withdrawal, as a preanesthetic medication, and in the treatment of status epilepticus

286. May cause increased alertness, elevated mood states, insomnia, irritability, and hallucinations

Questions 287–289

Many drugs are associated with an ability to induce physical dependence as well as a craving for and tolerance to their psychological effects. For each of the drugs listed below, choose the effect that it usually produces.

(A) Psychic dependence
(B) Tachyphylaxis
(C) Physical dependence only
(D) Tolerance and physical dependence
(E) Hallucinations
(F) Psychodelic effects
(G) Low potential of addiction

287. Meperidine

288. Secobarbital

289. Chlorpromazine

Central Nervous System
Answers

223. The answer is C. *(DiPalma, 3/e. pp 254–257, 266–272. Gilman, 8/e. pp 387–388, 396–397, 411.)* There are several chemical classes of compounds useful as antipsychotic agents. Phenothiazine derivatives (e.g., perphenazine) constitute the most numerous group and were the first antipsychotic drugs to be used. Thiothixene hydrochloride and chlorprothixene (Taractan) are two thiothixene derivatives used as antipsychotic drugs; butyrophenone derivatives are exemplified by haloperidol. Several other classes of heterocyclic compounds have antipsychotic activity, including loxapine succinate, molindone hydrochloride (Moban), and pimozide (Orap). Fluoxetine hydrochloride is a relatively new compound used as an antidepressant; it has no significant antipsychotic activity.

224. The answer is B. *(DiPalma, 3/e. p 307. Katzung, 4/e. p 374.)* Deaths have occurred from the administration of therapeutic doses of morphine to patients who had poor respiratory function such as in chronic cor pulmonale (pulmonary heart disease) or chronic obstructive pulmonary disease. Intravenous morphine can produce relief in dyspnea from acute pulmonary edema associated with left ventricular failure. For patients who have coronary artery disease, morphine can be beneficial because it decreases oxygen consumption and cardiac work. Morphine reduces the peristaltic contractions of the gastrointestinal tract and thus is useful in treating patients who have dysentery.

225. The answer is C. *(DiPalma, 3/e. pp 216–217.)* Triazolam is a benzodiazepine derivative, and like flurazepam and temazepam it is useful in the treatment of insomnia. It acts by binding to benzodiazepine receptors, enhancing GABA-mediated chloride influx. Adverse reactions include drowsiness, dizziness, lethargy, and ataxia. Though benzodiazepines alone do not significantly depress respiration, in combination with ethanol they can lead to severe respiratory depression. Unlike the barbiturates, benzodiazepines do not significantly induce the drug-metabolizing microsomal system at therapeutic doses.

226. The answer is E. *(DiPalma, 3/e. pp 274–276. Gilman, 8/e. pp 415–417.)* Phenelzine sulfate is a monoamine oxidase (MAO) inhibitor used for its antidepressant effects. The drug is irreversible and site-specific in that it inactivates the flavin prosthetic group of MAO following its oxidation to a reactive intermediate. The drug can produce orthostatic hypotension attributed to (1) enhanced stimulation of central alpha$_2$-adrenergic receptors leading to reduced sympathetic outflow, or (2) accumulation of octopamine, a false neurotransmitter, in sympathetic nerve terminals. Phenelzine can induce hypertensive crises when food containing high levels of tyramine, which stimulates the release of norepinephrine, is ingested. These foods include aged cheese, beer, wine, pickled herring, snails, chicken liver, yeast, citrus fruits, and chocolate. As opposed to the tricyclic antidepressants such as amitriptyline and nortriptyline, the monoamine oxidase inhibitors do not cause the cholinergic block that results in dry mouth, constipation, blurred vision, and urinary retention.

227. The answer is D. *(DiPalma, 3/e. pp 326, 332. Gilman, 8/e. p 321.)* Local anesthetics are agents that, when applied locally, block nerve conduction; they also prevent generation of a nerve impulse. All contain a lipophilic (benzene) functional group and most a hydrophilic (amine) group. Benzocaine does not contain the terminal hydrophilic amine group; thus, it is only slightly soluble in water and is slowly absorbed with a prolonged duration. It is, therefore, only useful as a surface anesthetic.

228. The answer is C. *(DiPalma, 3/e. pp 255–259. Katzung, 4/e. pp 348–349.)* Unwanted pharmacologic side effects produced by phenothiazine antipsychotic drugs (e.g., perphenazine) include Parkinson-like syndrome, akathisia, dystonias, galactorrhea, amenorrhea, and infertility. These side effects are due to the ability of these agents to block dopamine receptors. The phenothiazines also block muscarinic and alpha-adrenergic receptors, which are responsible for other effects.

229. The answer is D. *(DiPalma, 3/e. pp 326–328, 331.)* Mepivacaine is an amide-type local anesthetic. It acts by interfering with influx of sodium into nerve fibers. The drug has a moderately long duration of action (elimination half-life of 96 min). Mepivacaine is biotransformed in the liver; being an amide, it is not hydrolyzed by plasma esterases. Coadministration of epinephrine or levonordefrin (sympathomimetic amines) causes local vasoconstriction, thus prolonging the duration of action. Mepivacaine is not useful in obstetrics because of prolonged metabolism in the fetus and neonate, which increases the risk of toxicity. Adverse reactions caused by plasma buildup include CNS excitation followed by depression and cardiovascular depression.

230. The answer is D. *(DiPalma, 3/e. pp 159–160. Gilman, 8/e. pp 480–481.)* Malignant hyperthermia (hyperpyrexia), a syndrome associated with use of a general anesthetic (e.g., halothane) in conjunction with a skeletal muscle relaxant. is characterized by tachycardia, hyperventilation, arrhythmias, fever, muscular fasciculation, and rigidity. It is caused by a sudden increase in the availability of calcium ions in the myoplasma of muscle. Dantrolene, which interferes with release of calcium ions from the sarcoplasmic reticulum, is indicated in treatment of the disorder. The first three agents are centrally acting skeletal muscle relaxants that are not useful in the treatment of malignant hyperthermia.

231. The answer is D. *(AMA Drug Evaluations Annual 1991, 7/e. pp 239–242. Katzung, 4/e. pp 212–214.)* Mild analgesics such as aspirin and acetaminophen, sedatives, and antianxiety agents may provide nonspecific symptomatic relief for mild migraine headaches. Ergotamine is the most effective specific relief because of its vasoconstricting activity. Ergotamine is often combined with caffeine, which increases its oral absorption and also has cerebral vasoconstricting activity. Propranolol, a beta-adrenergic receptor blocker, and methysergide, a serotonergic receptor blocker, are useful in prophylactic therapy. Amitriptyline, a tricyclic antidepressant, and clonidine, an antihypertensive agent, have been used with some success in prophylactic therapy also.

232. The answer is C. *(DiPalma, 3/e. p 272. Gilman, 8/e. pp 405–406.)* The tricyclics and second-generation antidepressants act by blocking serotonin or norepinephrine uptake into the presynaptic terminal. Fluoxetine selectively inhibits serotonin uptake with minimal effects on norepinephrine uptake. Protriptyline, maprotiline, desipramine, and amoxapine have greater effect on norepinephrine uptake.

233. The answer is C. *(AMA Drug Evaluations Annual 1991, 7/e. pp 209–210. DiPalma, 3/e. pp 225–226.)* Some benzodiazepines are biotransformed to active products with CNS effects, some of which are long-lived. Desmethyldiazepam is a long-acting metabolite of chlordiazepoxide, clorazepate, alprazolam, diazepam, and prazepam. These compounds are more likely to produce cumulative effects and residual effects such as excessive drowsiness. Oxazepam and lorazepam are biotransformed to the inactive glucuronide.

234. The answer is C. *(DiPalma, 3/e. pp 256–259. Katzung, 4/e. pp 349–352.)* The phenothiazines (e.g., thioridazine) are antipsychotic agents. Autonomic manifestations result from alpha-adrenergic receptor and muscarinic cholinergic receptor blockade. A Parkinson-like syndrome results from blockade of dopaminergic receptors in the basal ganglia. Thioridazine has a lower incidence of acute extrapyramidal reactions than higher potency agents such as haloperidol and trifluoperazine. Chronic use of all these agents often leads to tardive dyskinesia. Although effective against vomiting produced by some drugs and disease states, phenothiazines are not effective for control of motion sickness. The phenothiazines block dopaminergic receptors in the pituitary, which subsequently increases secretion of prolactin, causing hyperprolactinemia and galactorrhea.

235. The answer is D. *(DiPalma, 3/e. pp 217–218. Gilman, 8/e. pp 364–365.)* Oral doses of chloral hydrate rapidly produce hypnosis and may cause epigastric distress, nausea, and vomiting. Although not biotransformed by the hepatic microsomal system, chloral hydrate accelerates the biotransformation of some drugs that are biotransformed by this system. Habitual use of chloral hydrate can lead to tolerance and physical dependence with delirium when the drug is withdrawn. Like the barbiturates, it has little analgesic activity and may produce excitement in the presence of pain.

236. The answer is E. *(DiPalma, 3/e. p 300. Katzung, 4/e. p 374.)* The extent and rate at which tolerance develops to the effects of opioid analgesics vary. A high degree of tolerance develops to analgesia, euphoria, sedation, respiratory depression, antidiuresis, nausea and vomiting, and cough suppression. A moderate degree develops to bradycardia. Little or no tolerance develops to the drug-induced miosis, constipation, and convulsions.

237. The answer is E. *(DiPalma, 3/e. pp 196, 203–204. Gilman, 8/e. pp 298–300.)* The large volume of nitrous oxide (N_2O) dissolved in the blood moves back into the alveoli by simple diffusion when administration of the gas is stopped. Thus, the alveolar concentration of oxygen may, temporarily, be markedly depressed. This situation is referred to as diffusion hypoxia and can cause postoperative hypoxemia.

238. The answer is C. *(DiPalma, 3/e. pp 288–290. Gilman, 8/e. p 471.)* Carbidopa is an inhibitor of aromatic L-amino acid decarboxylase. It cannot readily penetrate the CNS and thus decreases the decarboxylation of L-dopa in the peripheral tissues. This promotes an increased concentration of L-dopa in the nigrostriatum, where it is converted to dopamine. In addition, the effective dose of levodopa can be reduced.

239. The answer is E. *(DiPalma, 3/e. p 205. Katzung, 4/e. pp 312, 313.)* Ketamine is a dissociative anesthetic characterized by its ability to produce amnesia, analgesia, and catatonia. The compound may produce a gradual mild increase in muscle tone. It is the only intravenous anesthetic to routinely produce cardiovascular stimulation; the others may depress the heart rate and cardiac output.

240. The answer is D. *(DiPalma, 3/e. pp 273–274. Gilman, 8/e. pp 486–487.)* The enkephalins are endogenous agonists of the opioid receptors. They are located in areas of the brain and spinal cord related to the perception of pain. These areas include the laminae I and II of the spinal cord, the spinal trigeminal nucleus, and the periaqueductal gray. Selegiline and trihexyphenidyl are anti-parkinsonism drugs; baclofen is a skeletal muscle relaxant agonist for the GABA receptor.

241. The answer is B. *(Gilman, 8/e. p 459. Katzung, 4/e. pp 301–302.)* Intravenously administered diazepam is the drug of choice for treatment of status epilepticus. Diazepam increases the apparent affinity of the inhibitory neurotransmitter γ-aminobutyric acid (GABA) for binding sites on brain cell membranes. The effects of diazepam are short-lasting. Continuing therapy is usually with phenytoin. Other drugs suggested for use in status epilepticus are lorazepam and lidocaine. None of the other drugs listed in the question are appropriate for status epilepticus: chlorpromazine is an antipsychotic; succinylcholine is a neuromuscular blocking agent; tranylcypromine is an antidepressant; ethosuximide is used in petit mal epilepsy.

242. The answer is C. *(DiPalma, 3/e. pp 297–298, 301–302. Gilman, 8/e. pp 497, 504–506.)* Methadone is an opioid receptor agonist. It is used as an analgesic and to treat opioid abstinence and heroin users (methadone maintenance). The drug has greater oral efficacy than morphine and a much longer biologic half-life; this accounts for the milder but more protracted abstinence syndrome associated with methadone. Methadone does not possess opioid antagonist properties and thus would not precipitate withdrawal symptoms in a heroin addict, as would naloxone or naltrexone.

243. The answer is D. *(DiPalma, 3/e. pp 107–108. Gilman, 8/e. pp 189–190.)* Amphetamine is a noncatechol sympathomimetic amine that is a powerful CNS stimulant and can produce psychosis and hyperthermia. It is useful in the treatment of narcolepsy. In addition to its CNS stimulatory effects, the drug has peripheral sympathomimetic properties, leading to tachycardia, cardiac arrhythmias, anginal pain, and hypertension. Amphetamine is a mixed-acting agent that (1) stimulates release of norepinephrine, (2) inhibits monoamine oxidase, and (3) produces direct receptor stimulation. The methyl group on the alpha carbon makes the compound resistant to inactivation by monoamine oxidase. Since the phenyl ring does not contain hydroxyl groups in the 3,4 positions, amphetamine is not a catechol and, therefore, not metabolized by catechol-*O*-methyltransferase (COMT).

244. The answer is D. *(DiPalma, 3/e. pp 274–276.)* Tranylcypromine is a monoamine oxidase inhibitor, useful as an antidepressant. A second mode of action attributed to this agent is an amphetamine-like stimulant effect, which causes the release of norepinephrine. The tricyclic antidepressants inhibit uptake of serotonin or norepinephrine. Antipsychotics act by blocking dopamine receptors.

245. The answer is C. *(DiPalma, 3/e. pp 269, 273.)* Desipramine is a tricyclic antidepressant that acts primarily by inhibiting uptake of norepinephrine. Tricyclic antidepressants can produce many adverse reactions, including anticholinergic effects (e.g., xerostomia and constipation), sedation, orthostatic hypotension (partially owing to alpha-adrenergic blockade), tachycardia, and a decrease in REM sleep. Tricyclics also reduce the seizure threshold and can increase the risk of tonic-clonic seizures; they do not have anticonvulsant properties.

246. The answer is B. *(DiPalma, 3/e. p 204. Katzung, 4/e. pp 311–312.)* Thiopental is an intravenous general anesthetic. It is very useful for short procedures because it produces a rapid recovery, which is due to redistribution out of the brain. It produces little postanesthetic excitement or vomiting. Thiopental is biotransformed in the liver by desulfuration to pentobarbital. The compound can produce cough, laryngospasm, and bronchospasm. Thiopental, unlike halothane and related inhalation anesthetics, does *not* sensitize the myocardium to endogenous catecholamines.

247. The answer is B. *(DiPalma, 3/e. pp 235–236. Katzung, 4/e. pp 279–281.)* Ethanol is a central nervous system depressant. Among its many effects, it suppresses the release of antidiuretic hormone. Ethanol also causes peripheral vasodilation, particularly of cutaneous blood vessels. Though this may give one a feeling of warmth, heat is being dissipated and body temperature is lowered. Chronic use can lead to gastritis, pancreatitis, cirrhosis of the liver, and central effects such as Wernicke's encephalopathy and Korsakoff's psychosis. Acute overdose can lead to acidosis, hypoglycemia, and elevated intracranial pressure.

248. The answer is D. *(DiPalma, 3/e. p 230.)* Buspirone is an antianxiety agent not chemically related to the benzodiazepines. Though its exact mechanism of action is unknown, buspirone does not alter GABA receptors, but appears to have affinity for serotonin and dopamine (D_2) receptors. Buspirone lacks the anticonvulsant and skeletal muscle relaxant effects of the benzodiazepines and has minimal sedative effects. It does not produce the parkinsonian syndrome associated with antipsychotic drugs.

249. The answer is C. *(Katzung, 4/e. pp 335, 339.)* Two types of monoamine oxidase (MAO) have been found: MAO-A, which metabolizes norepinephrine and serotonin, and MAO-B, which metabolizes dopamine. Deprenyl (selegiline) is a selective inhibitor of MAO-B. It therefore inhibits the breakdown of dopamine and prolongs the therapeutic effectiveness of levodopa in parkinsonism. Bromocriptine is a dopamine receptor agonist. Carbidopa inhibits the peripheral metabolism of levodopa. Both are useful in treatment of parkinsonism. Phenelzine and tranylcypromine are nonselective MAO inhibitors. Combining them with levodopa may lead to hypertensive crises, and thus they are not used in the therapy of parkinsonism.

250. The answer is B. *(AMA Drug Evaluations Annual 1991, 7/e. pp 275–277.)* Based on its chemical structure, bupropion is classified as an atypical antidepressant drug. It has unique actions compared with other clinically effective antidepressant compounds. Bupropion has weak effects on norepinephrine and serotonin reuptake; however, it is an inhibitor of dopamine reuptake into dopaminergic neurons. Similar to the tricyclic antidepressants, the mechanism responsible for the antidepressant activity of bupropion is believed to be due to down-regulation of beta-adrenergic receptors in the CNS. In contrast to the tricyclic antidepressants, bupropion has no significant anticholinergic activity; additionally, it is not a monoamine oxidase inhibitor. Six biotransformation products have been identified, two of which have antidepressant activity (approximately half of that of the parent drug); however, following chronic administration of bupropion, these metabolites will accumulate so that the steady-state concentrations may reach up to 100 times that of bupropion itself.

Since the drug causes CNS stimulation, seizures have been noted in certain patients, e.g., those predisposed to seizures or those taking other drugs that lower the seizure threshold. It is suggested that the risk of seizures can be minimized by using lower total daily doses (i.e., 450 mg) than were originally tried and avoiding high peak concentrations of the drug by prescribing three divided doses rather than a large, single daily dose.

251. The answer is B. *(DiPalma, 3/e. pp 326–331. Katzung, 4/e. pp 315–319.)* Lidocaine is classified as an amide local anesthetic agent and has a rapid onset of action and excellent potency. It is a versatile agent useful in many clinical applications, such as surface anesthesia, peripheral nerve block, infiltration, and spinal and epidural anesthesia. Lidocaine may be combined with epinephrine to increase the former's duration of action. The vasoconstrictor effect of epinephrine will reduce the removal of lidocaine from its site of action. Lidocaine is biotransformed in the liver by amidases and undergoes *N*-dealkylation followed by sulfate conjugation.

252. The answer is D. *(AMA Drug Evaluations Annual 1991, 7/e. pp 199–231. DiPalma, 3/e. pp 225–229.)* Clorazepate is a benzodiazepine derivative, useful primarily as an antianxiety agent. The compound is inactive and must be hydrolyzed in the stomach to its active form. It can be further biotransformed in the liver; active metabolites include desmethyldiazepam and oxazepam. The metabolites have an elimination half-life of over 50 h. Prolonged use of benzodiazepines produces psychological and sometimes physical dependence.

253. The answer is C. *(DiPalma, 3/e. pp 300, 336–337. Gilman, 8/e. pp 495–504.)* In opioid abuse, there is always a high degree of cross tolerance to other drugs with a similar pharmacologic action even if the chemical composition of the opioids is totally different. Tolerance develops at different rates to different effects of opioids. With methadone, abrupt withdrawal causes a syndrome that is qualitatively similar to that of morphine but is longer and less intense, thus following the general rule that a drug with a shorter duration of action produces a shorter, more intense withdrawal syndrome. The crimes associated with narcotic abuse are considered to be motivated by the need to acquire the drug and not from the effects of the drug per se. Significant tolerance develops to most of the effects of narcotics except for constipation and pinpoint pupils, to which there is minimal tolerance.

254. The answer is D. *(AMA Drug Evaluations Annual 1991, 7/e. pp 201–205. DiPalma, 3/e. pp 216–217, 229.)* Indications for the benzodiazepines include anxiety and insomnia. Many, including chlordiazepoxide and diazepam, are used for anxiety. Flurazepam, temazepam, and triazolam are useful in the treatment of sleep disorders. Selected benzodiazepines are used in treatment of alcohol withdrawal (diazepam), seizure disorders (diazepam, clorazepate), nocturnal myoclonus (clonazepam), and skeletal muscle spasticity (diazepam). Lorazepam is useful intravenously as a premedication for endoscopic procedures or cardioversion. Chlordiazepoxide is classified as one of the long-acting benzodiazepines along with diazepam, prazepam, and clorazepate.

255. The answer is D. *(AMA Drug Evaluations Annual 1991, 7/e. p 242. Gilman, 8/e. p 399.)* Neuroleptic malignant syndrome is a condition characterized by hyperthermia, skeletal muscle hypertonicity, catatonia, elevated serum creatinine phosphokinase, fluctuations in consciousness, and labile heart rate and blood pressure. It is a relatively rare adverse reaction to potent antipsychotic drugs, such as trifluoperazine hydrochloride, especially when administered parenterally. Although the prevalence is estimated to be approximately 0.5 to 1 percent of those treated with antipsychotics, the mortality may be as high as 20 percent. This condition is treated by discontinuation of the antipsychotic drug and administration of dantrolene (Dantrium) intravenously (until the symptoms subside and the patient can swallow), then orally;

bromocriptine (Parlodel) is added to the therapy. This disorder has not been associated with antianxiety agents (e.g., oxazepam), sedative-hypnotics (e.g., amobarbital), antidepressants (e.g., doxepin hydrochloride), or antiepileptics (e.g., phenytoin).

256. The answer is B. *(AMA Drug Evaluations 1991, 7/e. p 349. Gilman, 8/e. p 475.)* Selegiline inhibits monoamine oxidase B, thus delaying the metabolic breakdown of dopamine. It is effective alone in parkinsonism and increases the effectiveness of levodopa. Benztropine and trihexyphenidyl are cholinergic agonists in the brain; bromocriptine is a dopamine receptor agonist. Chlorpromazine is an antipsychotic drug with antiadrenergic properties.

257. The answer is A. *(DiPalma, 3/e. pp 309–314, 431–436.)* Aspirin (acetylsalicylic acid), the most extensively used analgesic, antipyretic, and anti-inflammatory agent, acts generally by virtue of its salicylic acid content. Its therapeutic and adverse effects appear to be related to the degree of inhibition of the synthesis of prostaglandins. Aspirin is ulcerogenic to the gastrointestinal tract and inhibits platelet aggregation about equally to other salicylates. Acetaminophen, like aspirin, has analgesic and antipyretic properties but is not anti-inflammatory and is not irritating to the gastrointestinal tract.

258. The answer is A. *(AMA Drug Evaluations Annual 1991, 7/e. p 393. DiPalma, 3/e. p 258.)* Chlorpromazine is the prototype compound of the phenothiazine class of antipsychotic drugs. It is indicated for use in the treatment of a variety of psychoses, which includes schizophrenia, and in the treatment of nausea and vomiting, in both adults and children, from a number of causes. The drug can be administered orally, rectally, or intramuscularly for this purpose. It is believed that the effectiveness of the compound is based on inhibition of dopaminergic receptors in the chemoreceptor trigger zone of the medulla. Other phenothiazine derivatives are also used for emesis, including thiethylperazine (Torecan), prochlorperazine (Compazine), and perphenazine (Trilafon). Although chlorpromazine may cause orthostatic hypotension and has mild H_1-histamine receptor blocking activity, the drug is never used as an antihypertensive or as an antihistaminic. Chlorpromazine is not an effective antidepressant drug and lithium salts are used for treating the mania associated with bipolar affective disorder.

259. The answer is E. *(DiPalma, 3/e. pp 266, 270–273. Gilman, 8/e. pp 406–411.)* Maprotiline hydrochloride is a second-generation antidepressant, tetracyclic in structure. It acts by selectively blocking norepinephrine uptake into presynaptic nerve terminals; it has relatively weak activity on serotonin uptake and does not inhibit monoamine oxidase. Adverse reactions to this compound are similar to those of the tricyclic antidepressants, i.e., constipation, urinary hesitancy, blurred vision, sedation, and tachycardia. The autonomic adverse effects are due to blockade of muscarinic and alpha-adrenergic receptors.

260. The answer is A. *(DiPalma, 3/e. pp 297, 305. Gilman, 8/e. pp 512–513.)* Nalbuphine is a mixed opioid agonist-antagonist. It is an antagonist at μ receptors, a partial agonist at κ receptors, and an agonist at σ receptors. The drug is equipotent to morphine as an analgesic. Nalbuphine produces respiratory depression comparable to that of morphine at low-to-moderate doses. At higher doses there is a ceiling effect, with respiratory depression much less than that associated with morphine. Since nalbuphine is an antagonist at μ receptors, it can precipitate withdrawal in persons dependent on morphine or other μ agonists. In high doses the addiction potential is less than morphine and few cases of abuse have been reported.

261. The answer is A. *(DiPalma, 3/e. pp 263–265. Gilman, 8/e. pp 418–422.)* Lithium salts, such as lithium carbonate and lithium citrate, help to prevent the mania and to control mood swings in manic-depressive disorders. Unlike the phenothiazine derivatives, lithium is not a sedative; tremor is one of the most frequent adverse effects of lithium treatment. Renal toxicity includes lithium-induced nephrogenic diabetes insipidus and chronic interstitial nephritis during long-term therapy. Lithium also reduces thyroid function and produces edema. However, the use of diuretics to treat the lithium-induced edema will reduce the Na^+ concentrations in the body, which will promote the retention of lithium, thus increasing the potential toxicity of the drug. Since the safe and effective plasma concentration is considered to be between 0.75 and 1.25 meq/L, and concentrations above 2 meq/L have been associated with increased risk of more severe toxicity, the plasma concentrations of lithium should be monitored regularly.

262. The answer is D. *(DiPalma, 3/e. pp 248–250. Gilman, 8/e. pp 319–320.)* Cocaine has local anesthetic properties; it can block the initiation or conduction of a nerve impulse. It is biotransformed by plasma esterases to inactive products. In addition, cocaine blocks the reuptake of norepinephrine. This action produces CNS stimulant effects including euphoria, excitement, and restlessness. Peripherally, cocaine produces sympathomimetic effects including tachycardia and vasoconstriction. Death from acute overdose can be from respiratory depression or cardiac failure. Cocaine is an ester of benzoic acid and closely related to the structure of atropine.

263. The answer is D. *(DiPalma, 3/e. pp 281–288. Gilman, 8/e. pp 449–453.)* Both ethosuximide and valproic acid are used to treat absence seizures.

Ethosuximide is more effective than valproic acid for this purpose and exhibits fewer serious adverse effects. Valproic acid has been reported to cause hepatotoxicity. Carbamazepine is effective in the treatment of trigeminal neuralgia and all types of epilepsy except absence seizures. Phenobarbital and phenytoin are effective agents for generalized tonic-clonic and cortical focal seizures. Trimethadione, originally the special drug for absence seizures, is no longer the first choice because of its severe toxicity.

264. The answer is B. *(DiPalma, 3/e. pp 255–256. Katzung, 4/e. pp 338, 348.)* Central dopamine receptors are divided into D_1 and D_2 receptors. Antipsychotic activity is better correlated to blockade of D_2 receptors. Haloperidol, a potent antipsychotic, selectively antagonizes at D_2 receptors. Phenothiazine derivatives, such as chlorpromazine, fluphenazine, and promethazine, are not selective for D_2 receptors. Bromocriptine, a selective D_2 agonist, is useful in the treatment of parkinsonism and hyperprolactinemia. It produces fewer adverse reactions than do nonselective dopamine receptor agonists.

265. The answer is C. *(AMA Drug Evaluations Annual 1991, 7/e. pp 239–240, 353–354. Gilman, 8/e. p 404.)* Tourette's syndrome (or Gilles de la Tourette's syndrome) is manifested by severe motor tics and other involuntary movements, grunting, barking cries, and vocalizations that are frequently obscene. Most antipsychotic drugs are believed to be effective in treating this uncommon disorder; however, haloperidol is considered to be the drug of choice because of the large amount of clinical experience with this agent. Pimozide is an effective drug in Tourette's syndrome and should be considered for use when treatment with haloperidol has failed.

266. The answer is E. *(DiPalma, 3/e. pp 224–229, 254–256. Gilman, 8/e. pp 256–257.)* GABA is an inhibitory neurotransmitter that activates the chloride channel. Benzodiazepines, e.g., chlordiazepoxide and halazepam, bind to receptors on the chloride channel and enhance the binding of GABA to its receptor. Barbiturates also act on the chloride channel to increase the frequency of opening of the channel. Valproic acid elevates brain levels of GABA by inhibiting GABA metabolism. Chlorpromazine blocks the activity of dopamine receptors and has little or no effect on the GABA system.

267. The answer is E. *(DiPalma, 3/e. pp 243–244, 250–253. Gilman, 8/e. pp 550–551.)* The active ingredient in marijuana is Δ^9-tetrahydrocannabinol. In general, marijuana is a CNS stimulant causing tachycardia, giddiness, and, at high doses, visual hallucinations. Acute intoxication is characterized by reddening of the conjunctiva (bloodshot eyes) owing to local vasodilation. Potential therapeutic uses include antiemesis in cancer chemotherapy and reduction of intraocular pressure in glaucoma. Chronic use has been associated with an "amotivational syndrome" and with a reduction in serum testosterone and sperm count. Flashbacks are a major symptom of use of lysergic acid diethylamide (LSD).

268. The answer is D. *(DiPalma, 3/e. pp 336–339. Gilman, 8/e. pp 366, 531–539.)* Physical dependence occurs following prolonged use of morphine, ethanol, barbiturates, and nonbarbiturates such as glutethimide. Acute withdrawal of these substances produces an abstinence syndrome, the severity of which depends upon the drug. Withdrawal of cocaine after chronic use can lead to craving for the drug, prolonged sleep, general fatigue, lassitude, hyperphagia, and depression. This meets the criteria for a withdrawal syndrome.

269. The answer is D. *(DiPalma, 3/e. pp 306–307. Katzung, 4/e. p 381.)* Naltrexone and naloxone are pure opioid antagonists with no agonist activity at therapeutic doses. In opioid-dependent persons, these agents will precipitate withdrawal syndrome. Naltrexone is much better absorbed from the gastrointestinal tract and is useful by oral administration. It also has a much longer duration of action, making it useful in treatment programs for drug addicts. Although naltrexone does have a "first-pass" effect in the liver, the metabolic product is also active.

270. The answer is C. *(DiPalma, 3/e. pp 315–320. Gilman, 8/e. pp 656–659.)* All the drugs mentioned with the exception of acetaminophen achieve their therapeutic and toxic effects by inhibition of prostaglandin synthesis. The group includes salicylates as well as sulindac and fenoprofen and is known as nonsteroidal anti-inflammatory drugs (NSAIDS). Acetaminophen is equal in analgesic potency to NSAIDS but has no effect on prostaglandins. It is also nonulcerogenic—a great advantage in patients who are ulcer-prone.

271. The answer is B. *(DiPalma, 3/e. pp 234, 236–237. Gilman, 8/e. pp 376, 526.)* Chronic consumption of ethanol causes hypertrophy of the hepatic smooth endoplasmic reticulum with a resultant increase in metabolic enzymes. The induction of the microsomal system may play a role in the enhanced biotransformation of ethanol and, thus, the development of metabolic or dispositional tolerance. Barbiturates are biotransformed via the microsomal system; however, in the presence of ethanol, which is preferentially metabolized, barbiturates remain active longer. Symptoms of ethanol withdrawal can include restlessness, insomnia, tremors, disorientation, hallucinations, and convulsions. Chronic effects of ethanol abuse may include gastritis, pancreatitis, hepatitis, cirrhosis of the liver, and cardiomegaly.

272. The answer is B. *(DiPalma, 3/e. pp 212–215. Gilman, 8/e. pp 358–364.)* The termination of the action of ultra-short-acting barbiturates such as methohexital and thiopental is due to redistribution of the drugs from the brain. Following redistribution thiopental is biotransformed to pentobarbital, which is further oxidized to inactive products. Chronic administration of barbiturates can induce enzymes in the liver. Barbiturates are contraindicated in acute intermittent porphyria because they increase δ-aminolevulinic acid, which produces an elevation of porphyrins in the body. In patients with acute intermittent porphyria, the precipitous increase of porphyrins may result in paralysis and death. All barbiturates possess anticonvulsant activity, but only phenobarbital, mephobarbital, and metharbital have antiepileptic properties. These drugs may be used in the treatment of tonic-clonic seizures, psychomotor seizures, and other types of epilepsy. Although alkalinization of the urine may promote the excretion of weak acidic drugs such as the barbiturates, it appears that only the excretion of phenobarbital is enhanced by increasing the pH of the urine. In the renal tubular fluid phenobarbital is converted more to the anionic form, and this form of phenobarbital is not readily reabsorbed by the renal tubular cells.

273. The answer is B. *(DiPalma, 3/e. p 302. Gilman, 8/e. pp 508–517.)* The synthetic opioid fentanyl is 80 to 100 times more potent than morphine and has a major use in anesthesia. It is combined with droperidol, an antipsychotic butyrophenone, to produce neuroleptanalgesia. Muscular rigidity produced by fentanyl very likely results from opioid influence on dopaminergic transmission in the striatum, an influence that is antagonized by naloxone. Fentanyl is only available as an injection to be used intravenously in anesthesia.

274. The answer is B. *(DiPalma, 3/e. pp 196, 198–201. Gilman, 8/e. pp 286–292.)* The high solubility of halothane, a halogenated alkane, in blood and fat allows for the maintenance of anesthetic blood levels for prolonged periods. The death rate associated with halothane is similar to or slightly lower than that of other anesthetic agents. Halothane is a very potent anesthetic (MAC = 0.75) compared with nitrous oxide (MAC = 105). Hepatotoxicity does occasionally occur and appears to increase in incidence with increased exposure to halothane. Depression of respiratory centers expressed as a decreased ventilatory response to carbon dioxide occurs as anesthetic depth increases. Arterial hypotension and a reduction in cardiac output, peripheral resistance, and myocardial contractility occur at surgical levels of anesthesia.

275. The answer is E. *(DiPalma, 3/e. pp 288–291. Gilman, 8/e. pp 466–475.)* Drugs useful in the therapy of parkinsonism act through several mechanisms. Levodopa, primary therapy for parkinsonism, is the immediate precursor to dopamine and thus increases brain levels of dopamine by enhancing its synthesis. Benztropine is one of several muscarinic blocking agents and is a useful adjunct in therapy. Amantadine, an antiviral agent, acts by stimulating release of dopamine from storage sites. Bromocriptine is a direct agonist at dopaminergic receptors. Selegiline, a relatively new drug, selectively inhibits monoamine oxidase B, which is present in the brain. Monoamine oxidase A is located mainly in the liver and the gut.

276. The answer is D. *(AMA Drug Evaluations Annual 1991, 7/e. p 58. DiPalma, 3/e. pp 297–301.)* Codeine is an opioid analgesic useful in relieving mild-to-moderate pain. Its effects are qualitatively similar to those of morphine, but it is a less potent analgesic. It is also useful by oral administration as an antitussive agent. Adverse reactions to codeine include (1) respiratory depression, which is reversed by naloxone; (2) hypotension, cutaneous vasodilation, and urticaria, which are a result of histamine release; and (3) constipation. Codeine is biotransformed in the liver, partially by demethylation to morphine. Codeine is as addictive as other opiates and is under control of the Drug Enforcement Administration (DEA).

277. The answer is D. *(DiPalma, 3/e. pp 297, 306–307. Gilman, 8/e. p 488.)* Naloxone is a pure opioid antagonist at μ, κ, and σ receptors. It will reverse the analgesic and other opioid effects of agonists (e.g., morphine) and agonist-antagonists (e.g., butorphanol). Naloxone will also induce withdrawal in an opioid (heroin) addict. Though naloxone will reverse opioid-induced respiratory depression, it is not effective in reversing phenobarbital-induced respiratory depression. The drug is only useful by injection for emergency treatment of opioid overdose. Naltrexone, another opioid antagonist, is useful orally for treatment of drug addiction.

278. The answer is C. *(DiPalma, 3/e. pp 225–229.)* Alprazolam is a benzodiazepine derivative classified as an antianxiety agent. It acts by potentiating the activity of GABA. On a weight basis, it is the most potent antianxiety agent. Of the benzodiazepines, only diazepam is useful in relief of skeletal muscle spasm. The benzodiazepines, administered orally, produce only mild respiratory depression; barbiturates have significant depressant effects. Combining benzodiazepines with other CNS depressants (e.g., ethanol) can cause significant respiratory depression.

279. The answer is B. *(DiPalma, 3/e. pp 339–340.)* "Crack" is the free-base form (nonsalt form) of the alkaloid cocaine. It is called crack because when heated it makes a crackling sound. Heating crack enables a person to smoke it; the drug is readily absorbed through the lungs and produces an intense euphoric effect in seconds. Use has led to seizures and cardiac arrhythmias. Some of cocaine's effects (sympathomimetic) are due to blockade of norepinephrine reuptake into presynaptic terminals; it does not block receptors. "Flashbacks" can occur with use of LSD and mescaline but have not been associated with the use of cocaine.

280. The answer is B. *(DiPalma, 3/e. pp 245–246. Gilman, 8/e. pp 557–558.)* Acute overdose of phencyclidine, a psychotomimetic agent, results in anxiety, agitation, aggression, and hallucinations. Severe overdose may lead to dysphoria, catatonia, muscle rigidity, convulsions, hypertensive crises, delirium, and coma. Autonomic effects include tachycardia, diaphoresis, sweating, salivation, and lacrimation. Treatment is symptomatic. Vital signs are supported, urine is acidified, and gastric suction may be performed (phencyclidine has a high gastroenteric recirculation). Parenteral diazepam and an antihypertensive should be given. Haloperidol or a phenothiazine may be used to treat psychosis. Propranolol is used in controlling excessive sympathetic stimulation.

281–283. The answers are: 281-E, 282-K, 283-I. *(AMA Drug Evaluations Annual 1991, 7/e. pp 235, 248–249, 252–253, 262–263, 268–271. DiPalma, 3/e. pp 268–269. Gilman, 8/e. pp 396–397.)* Amitriptyline is one of the oldest of the tricyclic antidepressants. Both amitriptyline and doxepin (Sinequan) are quite sedating and have the greatest anticholinergic activity of all the many tricyclic antidepressants available. Biotransformation by *N*-demethylation results in the production of the active metabolite, nortriptyline (which is also available for use in the treatment of depression as Aventyl).

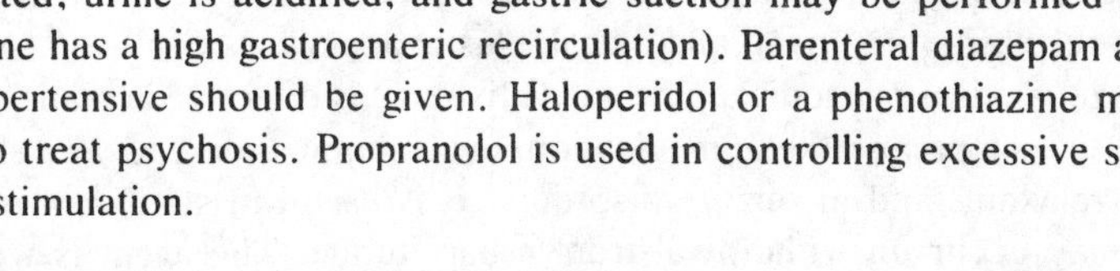

Amitriptyline　　　　Nortriptyline

Fluphenazine enanthate and fluphenazine decanoate are available for use as depot injections; these preparations have a duration of action of 1 to 4 weeks and are useful for patients with a history of poor compliance, or those with an inadequate absorption of oral medications. Haloperidol, as the decanoate salt (Haldol Decanoate), is also available for depot intramuscular injection and is usually given once every 3 to 4 weeks.

Clozapine is a low-potency drug that appears to be beneficial for use in severely ill patients who have failed to respond adequately to other antipsychotic agents. The pharmacology of this compound is atypical as compared with other antipsychotics in that it has weak dopaminergic potency, but it may alter dopaminergic function at higher centers in the brain than do other drugs. The incidence of extrapyramidal reactions (i.e., Parkinson-like symptoms and tardive dyskinesia) and elevation of prolactin concentrations are minimal. However, the most severe toxicity is the rather high incidence of agranulocytosis (approximately 1 percent); this requires that patients have regular (weekly is recommended) white blood cell counts.

284–286. The answers are: 284-G, 285-L, 286-C. *(DiPalma, 3/e. pp 108, 225–229, 282–283, 402. Gilman, 8/e. pp 211–212, 441–442.)* Phenytoin is one of the most commonly used antiepileptic agents. Chronic administration has been reported to cause such adverse reactions as ataxia, dizziness, nystagmus, gingival hyperplasia, hirsutism, and megaloblastic anemia.

Diazepam is a benzodiazepine derivative and is effective in management of anxiety, as a preanesthetic medication, in alcohol withdrawal, as a skeletal muscle relaxant, and in seizure disorders. It is useful in status epilepticus, which may occur on withdrawal from a barbiturate. The agent is well absorbed orally, is highly protein-bound (greater than 90 percent), and is biotransformed in the liver to active products. Flurazepam and triazolam are benzodiazepine derivatives that are used exclusively as hypnotics.

Dextroamphetamine, a mixed-acting adrenergic drug, is more potent than the *l* isomer in producing CNS stimulation. Some central nervous system effects of use of dextroamphetamine may be increased alertness, elevated mood states, insomnia, irritability, dizziness, violent behavior, and hallucination. Although phenylephrine is an adrenergic agonist, its central stimulatory effects are minimal.

287–289. The answers are: 287-D, 288-D, 289-G. *(DiPalma, 3/e. pp 334–341. Katzung, 4/e. pp 383–390.)* Heroin and other opioids (such as morphine and meperidine) exhibit a high degree of tolerance and physical dependence. The magnitudes of rates of tolerance to all the effects of opioids are not necessarily the same. The physical dependence is quite clear from the character and severity of withdrawal symptoms, which include vomiting spasms, abdominal cramps, diarrhea, and acid-base imbalances among others.

Secobarbital exhibits the same pharmacologic properties as other members of the barbiturate class. While there may be considerable tolerance to the sedative and intoxicating effects of the drug, the lethal dose is not much greater in addicted than normal persons. Severe withdrawal symptoms in epileptic patients may include grand mal seizures and delirium.

No current evidence exists that chlorpromazine, an antipsychotic agent, is addicting. Although some tolerance and physical dependence have been suggested. the failure to detect any EEG changes upon abrupt cessation of the drug implies that these effects are not of major importance.

None of these drugs have significant association with hallucinations or psychedelic effects. Lysergic acid diethylamide (LSD) is the primary agent deemed to possess these attributes.

Autonomic Nervous System

- General Considerations
  - Anatomic
  - Physiologic
  - Nature of synaptic transmission
  - Cholinergic transmission
  - Adrenergic transmission
  - Receptors, adrenergic and cholinergic
- Adrenergic Drugs
  - Sites and mode of action
  - Chemistry and structure-activity relationships
  - Direct-acting agonists
    - Epinephrine*
    - Norepinephrine*
    - Isoproterenol*
    - Phenylephrine
    - Dobutamine
    - Terbutaline
    - Albuterol*
    - Metaproterenol
    - Isoetharine
    - Ritodrine
    - Tetrahydrozoline
  - Indirect-acting agents
    - Tyramine*
  - Mixed-acting agents
    - Dopamine*
    - Ephedrine*
    - Phenylpropanolamine
    - Amphetamines
    - Pseudoephedrine
- Beta-Adrenergic Blocking Drugs
  - Propranolol*
  - Acebutolol
  - Atenolol
  - Betaxolol
  - Esmolol
  - Labetalol
  - Metoprolol
  - Nadolol
  - Pindolol
  - Timolol
- Alpha-Adrenergic Blocking Drugs
  - Nonselective
    - Phentolamine*
    - Phenoxybenzamine*
    - Ergot alkaloids, ergonovine, ergotamine
  - Selective
    - Prazosin,* terazosin, doxazosin
    - Yohimbine
- Adrenergic Neuronal Blocking Drugs
  - Reserpine*
  - Guanethidine,* guanadrel
  - Metyrosine
- Cholinomimetic Agents
  - Direct-acting
    - Choline esters
      - Acetylcholine*
      - Methacholine
      - Carbachol
      - Bethanechol
    - Naturally occurring muscarinic alkaloids
      - Muscarine*
      - Pilocarpine*
    - Naturally occurring nicotinic alkaloids
      - Nicotine*
      - Lobeline

- Indirect Acting
  - Reversible cholinesterase inhibitors
    - Physostigmine*
    - Neostigmine
    - Pyridostigmine
    - Edrophonium
    - Ambenomium chloride
  - Irreversible cholinesterase inhibitors
    - Isoflurophate*
    - Echothiophate iodide
    - Malathion*
    - Soman, sarin, tabun
- Antidotes for Organophosphate Poisoning
  - Atropine
  - Pralidoxime chloride
- Antimuscarinic Drugs
  - Atropine*
  - Homatropine*
  - Scopolamine*
  - Propantheline bromide
  - Cyclopentolate
  - Tropicamide
  - Anisotropine
  - Ipratropium
  - Methscopolamine
  - Trihexyphenidyl*
- Ganglionic Blocking Drugs
  - Mecamylamine
  - Trimethaphan camsylate
  - Nicotine
- Skeletal-Muscle Relaxants
  - Neuromuscular blocking agents
    - Depolarizing drugs
      - Succinylcholine*
    - Nondepolarizing drugs
      - Tubocurarine*
      - Metocurine
      - Gallamine
      - Pancuronium
      - Vecuronium
      - Atracurium
  - Centrally acting skeletal-muscle relaxants
    - Baclofen
    - Cyclobenzaprine
    - Diazepam
  - Direct-acting skeletal-muscle relaxant
    - Dantrolene
- MAO Inhibitors
  - Selegiline*
  - Tranylcypromine
  - Isocarboxazid
  - Phenelzine

DIRECTIONS: Each question below contains five suggested responses. Select the **one best** response to each question.

290. The alpha-adrenergic receptor antagonist that produces an irreversible, nonequilibrium receptor blockade is

(A) phentolamine (Regitine)
(B) phenoxybenzamine (Dibenzyline)
(C) prazosin (Minipress)
(D) terazosin (Hytrin)
(E) ergotamine (Ergomar)

291. All the following are possible effects of low doses of nicotine (from smoking tobacco products) EXCEPT

(A) increased tone and motor activity of the intestine
(B) stimulation of respiratory rate and depth
(C) stimulation of catecholamine release from the adrenal medulla
(D) bradycardia
(E) nausea and vomiting

292. All the following drugs have significant antimuscarinic effects EXCEPT

(A) diphenhydramine (Benadryl)
(B) pyridostigmine (Mestinon)
(C) meperidine (Demerol)
(D) amitriptyline (Elavil)
(E) thioridazine (Mellaril)

293. Epinephrine and norepinephrine must be given parenterally to elicit systemic effects. All the following are reasons these drugs are ineffective orally EXCEPT

(A) because of their low lipid solubility, these compounds are poorly absorbed following oral administration
(B) both drugs complex with divalent cations found in digestive secretions that prevent their transfer across the intestinal mucosa
(C) these drugs are inactivated by enzymes found in the digestive secretions
(D) both compounds produce a local vasoconstrictor effect that reduces blood flow and absorption through the gastrointestinal mucosa
(E) these catecholamines are rapidly inactivated by enzymes in the intestinal mucosa and liver

294. The enzyme that is inhibited by echothiophate iodide (Phospholine Iodide) is

(A) tyrosine hydroxylase
(B) acetylcholinesterase
(C) catechol-*O*-methyltransferase
(D) monoamine oxidase
(E) carbonic anhydrase

295. A 24-year-old man is brought to the emergency room by a group of friends who said that he had suddenly become restless, confused, and uncoordinated after taking some pills. Physical examination reveals increased body temperature, tachycardia, cutaneous flush, and widely dilated pupils unresponsive to light. The patient complains of dryness of the mouth. He probably ingested which of the following drugs?

(A) Codeine
(B) Aspirin
(C) Secobarbital
(D) Atropine
(E) Chlordiazepoxide

296. All the following statements are true concerning isoproterenol (Isuprel) EXCEPT that

(A) it is readily absorbed when administered parenterally or by aerosol
(B) it lowers peripheral resistance and diastolic blood pressure
(C) it relaxes bronchial smooth muscle
(D) it is biotransformed primarily in the liver by monoamine oxidase (MAO)
(E) it is used as a cardiac stimulant in heart block and cardiogenic shock after myocardial infarction

297. The nonselective beta-adrenergic blocking agent that is also a competitive antagonist at $alpha_1$-adrenoceptors is

(A) timolol (Blocadren)
(B) nadolol (Corgard)
(C) pindolol (Visken)
(D) acebutolol (Sectral)
(E) labetalol (Normodyne)

298. All the following are effects of serotonin (5-hydroxytryptamine) EXCEPT

(A) relaxation of gastrointestinal smooth muscle
(B) vasoconstriction of arterioles of the pulmonary and renal beds
(C) bronchoconstriction
(D) stimulation of pain and itching
(E) vasodilation of arterioles in the heart and skeletal muscle

299. Propranolol (Inderal) is either contraindicated in, or should be used with caution in, all the following disease states EXCEPT

(A) hypoglycemia
(B) Raynaud's phenomenon
(C) bronchial asthma
(D) congestive heart failure
(E) angina pectoris

300. All the following structures respond to beta-adrenergic receptor stimulation EXCEPT

(A) the ciliary muscle of the iris
(B) the radial muscle of the iris
(C) bronchial muscle
(D) the atrioventricular node
(E) the sinoatrial node

301. All the following drugs act within sympathetic neurons to depress neurotransmitter release and are used to treat hypertension EXCEPT

(A) guanadrel (Hylorel)
(B) metyrosine (Demser)
(C) selegiline (Eldepryl)
(D) reserpine (Serpasil)
(E) guanethidine (Ismelin)

302. All the following statements are true concerning the use of dopamine (Intropin) EXCEPT

(A) this drug must be given by intravenous infusion since it is rapidly biotransformed
(B) small doses of dopamine cause an increase in glomerular filtration rate, renal blood flow, and Na^+ excretion
(C) at intermediate concentrations, the administration of dopamine results in a positive inotropic effect on the myocardium
(D) high concentrations of dopamine cause vasoconstriction, increased peripheral vascular resistance, and elevation of mean blood pressure
(E) central nervous system adverse effects (including sedation, lethargy, and depression) are commonly experienced by patients during the administration of the drug

303. In certain patients, the duration of apnea produced after administration of succinylcholine is hours rather than a few minutes. These patients probably have a deficiency of

(A) liver transglycosylase
(B) liver hydroxymethylase
(C) plasma cholinesterase
(D) plasma glycine transamidinase
(E) red blood cell glucose-6-phosphate dehydrogenase

304. Atropine and scopolamine will block all the effects of acetylcholine listed below EXCEPT

(A) bradycardia
(B) salivary secretion
(C) bronchoconstriction
(D) skeletal muscle contraction
(E) miosis

305. All the following statements are true for both terbutaline (Brethine) and isoetharine (Bronkosol) EXCEPT

(A) these drugs are direct-acting, selective beta$_2$-adrenergic receptor agonists
(B) both compounds will increase adenylate cyclase activity in bronchiolar smooth muscle
(C) extensive first-pass biotransformation of these drugs will occur following oral administration
(D) both compounds can be given by inhalation or orally for the treatment of bronchospasm
(E) two common adverse effects associated with these drugs are muscle tremors and tachycardia

306. Propranolol (Inderal) is indicated for use in patients with all the following conditions EXCEPT

(A) hypertension
(B) angina pectoris
(C) glaucoma
(D) migraine headaches
(E) supraventricular and ventricular arrhythmias

307. Phenylephrine (Neo-Synephrine), which is included in over-the-counter cold remedies,

(A) causes vasoconstriction by stimulation of alpha-adrenergic receptors
(B) prevents vasodilation by blocking beta-adrenergic receptors
(C) stimulates the central nervous system to increase blood flow
(D) reduces secretion by inhibiting parasympathetic stimulation
(E) is an antihistamine that reduces secretion

308. Hypotension, bradycardia, respiratory depression, and muscle weakness, all unresponsive to atropine and neostigmine, would most likely be due to

(A) diazoxide
(B) isoflurophate
(C) tubocurarine
(D) nicotine
(E) pilocarpine

309. Ritodrine hydrochloride (Yutopar) is used in the treatment of

(A) Parkinson's disease
(B) bronchial asthma
(C) depression
(D) hypertension
(E) premature labor

310. The skeletal muscle relaxant that acts directly on the contractile mechanism of the muscle fibers is

(A) gallamine (Flaxedil)
(B) baclofen (Lioresal)
(C) pancuronium (Pavulon)
(D) cyclobenzaprine (Flexeril)
(E) dantrolene (Dantrium)

311. A predictably dangerous side effect of nadolol (Corgard) that constitutes a contraindication to its clinical use in susceptible patients is the induction of

(A) hypertension
(B) cardiac arrhythmia
(C) asthmatic attacks
(D) respiratory depression
(E) hypersensitivity

312. All the following drugs are used topically in the treatment of chronic wide-angle glaucoma. Which of these agents reduces intraocular pressure by decreasing the formation of the aqueous humor?

(A) Betaxolol hydrochloride (Betoptic)
(B) Echothiophate iodide (Phospholine Iodide)
(C) Pilocarpine hydrochloride (Pilocar)
(D) Isoflurophate (Floropryl)
(E) Physostigmine salicylate (Isopto Eserine)

313. The cholinomimetic drug that is useful for treating postoperative abdominal distention and gastric atony is

(A) acetylcholine (Miochol)
(B) methacholine (Provocholine)
(C) carbachol (Isopto Carbachol)
(D) bethanechol (Urecholine)
(E) pilocarpine (Pilocar)

314. Neostigmine (Prostigmin) will effectively antagonize skeletal muscle relaxation produced by

(A) metocurine (Metubine)
(B) succinylcholine (Anectine)
(C) diazepam (Valium)
(D) baclofen (Lioresal)
(E) nicotine (Nicorette)

315. All the following statements are true concerning the use of therapeutic oral doses of amphetamine EXCEPT

(A) the drug may cause hypotension by decreasing both systolic and diastolic blood pressure
(B) wakefulness, alertness, headache, and agitation are common CNS effects of the drug
(C) anorexia is a common effect of this drug
(D) narcolepsy and attention-deficit hyperactivity disorder are approved indications for amphetamine
(E) amphetamine induces the release of biogenic amines from storage sites in neuron terminals

316. All the following drugs can produce bronchodilation and are indicated for the therapy of bronchial asthma EXCEPT

(A) theophylline
(B) isoproterenol
(C) tetrahydrozoline
(D) albuterol
(E) aminophylline

317. The mechanism of action of the long-lasting organic phosphate anticholinesterases is

(A) splitting of polypeptide bonds in cholinesterases
(B) phosphorylation of the anionic site of cholinesterases
(C) phosphorylation of the esteratic site of cholinesterases
(D) acetylation of the anionic site of cholinesterases
(E) acetylation of the esteratic site of cholinesterases

318. Pralidoxime chloride (Protopam Chloride) is a drug that

(A) reduces the vesicular stores of catecholamines in adrenergic and dopaminergic neurons
(B) blocks the active transport of choline into cholinergic neurons
(C) reactivates cholinesterases that have been inhibited by organophosphate cholinesterase inhibitors
(D) stimulates the activity of phospholipase C with increased formation of inositol triphosphate
(E) inhibits the reuptake of biogenic amines into nerve terminals

319. Which of the following antimuscarinic drugs is used by inhalation in the treatment of bronchial asthma?

(A) Anisotropine methylbromide (Valpin)
(B) Cyclopentolate hydrochloride (Cyclogyl)
(C) Ipratropium bromide (Atrovent)
(D) Methscopolamine bromide (Pamine)
(E) Trihexyphenidyl hydrochloride (Artane)

320. All the following statements are accurate characterizations of ephedrine EXCEPT that it

(A) is used as a decongestant
(B) can cause insomnia, restlessness, agitation, and tremors
(C) can increase systemic blood pressure
(D) is rapidly biotransformed by both catechol-*O*-methyltransferase (COMT) and monamine oxidase (MAO)
(E) will relax the smooth muscles of the bronchial tree

321. The cholinesterase inhibitor that is used in the diagnosis of myasthenia gravis is

(A) edrophonium chloride (Tensilon)
(B) ambenonium chloride (Mytelase)
(C) malathion
(D) physostigmine salicylate (Antilirium)
(E) pyridostigmine bromide (Mestinon)

322. All the following are possible effects of mecamylamine (Inversine) EXCEPT

(A) arteriolar vasodilatation
(B) mydriasis and cycloplegia
(C) constipation and urinary retention
(D) tachycardia
(E) skeletal muscle weakness

323. Epinephrine may be mixed with certain anesthetics, such as procaine, in order to

(A) stimulate local wound repair
(B) promote hemostasis
(C) enhance their interaction with neural membranes and their ability to depress nerve conduction
(D) retard their systemic absorption
(E) facilitate their distribution along nerves and fascial planes

324. All the following drugs block beta$_1$-adrenergic receptors in the heart EXCEPT

(A) propranolol (Inderal)
(B) metoprolol (Lopressor)
(C) haloperidol (Haldol)
(D) atenolol (Tenormin)
(E) esmolol (Brevibloc)

325. Cyproheptadine (Periactin) is an antagonist at

(A) histamine (H_2) receptors
(B) dopamine (D_1) receptors
(C) serotonin (5-HT) receptors
(D) nicotine (N2) receptors
(E) norepinephrine (alpha) receptors

326. All the following statements are true concerning dobutamine hydrochloride (Dobutrex) EXCEPT that it

(A) is a selective agonist at $beta_1$-adrenergic receptors
(B) activates dopaminergic receptors in renal and mesenteric vascular beds
(C) is used to increase cardiac output in patients with severe cardiac failure
(D) must be given by intravenous administration
(E) may cause tachycardia and anginal pain

327. The skeletal muscles that are most sensitive to the action of tubocurarine are the

(A) muscles of the trunk
(B) muscles of the arms and legs
(C) respiratory muscles
(D) muscles of the head, neck, and face
(E) abdominal muscles

328. Which of the following is used in the treatment of acute migraine headaches because of its vasoconstrictor properties?

(A) Ergotamine
(B) Propranolol
(C) Methysergide
(D) Pseudoephedrine
(E) Aspirin

329. All the following are effects elicited by activation of the parasympathetic nervous system EXCEPT

(A) decreased heart rate
(B) increased tone of longitudinal smooth muscles of the intestine
(C) contraction of skeletal muscles
(D) contraction of the detrusor of the urinary bladder
(E) secretion of fluid from the lacrimal glands

330. The drug of choice for the treatment of anaphylactic shock is

(A) epinephrine
(B) norepinephrine
(C) isoproterenol
(D) diphenhydramine
(E) atropine

331. Both phentolamine (Regitine) and prazosin (Minipress)

(A) are competitive antagonists at $alpha_1$-adrenergic receptors
(B) have potent direct vasodilator actions on vascular smooth muscle
(C) enhance gastric acid secretion via a histamine-like effect
(D) cause hypotension and bradycardia
(E) are used chronically for the treatment of primary hypertension

332. Pancuronium bromide (Pavulon) may cause an increased heart rate due to

(A) a reflex response to hypotension caused by the drug
(B) blockade of N1 receptors in parasympathetic ganglia
(C) its vagolytic action on the heart
(D) a digitalis-like action on the myocardium
(E) direct stimulation of the vasomotor center in the brainstem

333. All the following compounds are believed to function as cotransmitters or neuromodulators that exist with acetylcholine or norepinephrine in neurons of the autonomic nervous system EXCEPT

(A) vasoactive intestinal peptide (VIP)
(B) adenosine triphosphate (ATP)
(C) neuropeptide Y (NPY)
(D) substance P
(E) serotonin (5-HT)

DIRECTIONS: Each group of questions below consists of lettered headings followed by a set of numbered items. For each numbered item, select the **one** lettered heading with which it is **most** closely associated. Each lettered heading may be used **once, more than once, or not at all.**

Questions 334–337

For each pharmacologic action listed, select the drug with which it is most likely to be associated.

(A) Diazepam (Valium)
(B) Doxazosin (Cardura)
(C) Scopolamine (Transderm Scop)
(D) Cyclobenzaprine hydrochloride (Flexeril)
(E) Propantheline bromide (Pro-Banthine)
(F) Atracurium besylate (Tracrium)
(G) Atenolol (Tenormin)
(H) Baclofen (Lioresal)
(I) Timolol maleate (Timoptic)
(J) Phentolamine mesylate (Regitine)

334. Reduces intraocular pressure

335. Blocks muscarinic receptors in the periphery and central nervous system

336. Causes skeletal muscle paralysis

337. Selective $alpha_1$-adrenergic antagonist

Questions 338–340

For each anatomic site listed, select the catecholamine neurotransmitter found in the highest amounts.

(A) Dopamine
(B) Serotonin
(C) Epinephrine
(D) Norepinephrine
(E) Acetylcholine

338. Adrenergic fibers

339. Adrenal medulla

340. Caudate nucleus

Questions 341–344

The figure below illustrates proposed sites of action of drugs. For each drug listed, select the site of action that the drug is most likely to *inhibit*. (α = alpha receptor; β = beta receptor; COMT = catechol-*O*-methyltransferase; MAO = monoamine oxidase; NE = norepinephrine; NMN = normetanephrine)

SYMPATHETIC NEUROEFFECTOR JUNCTION

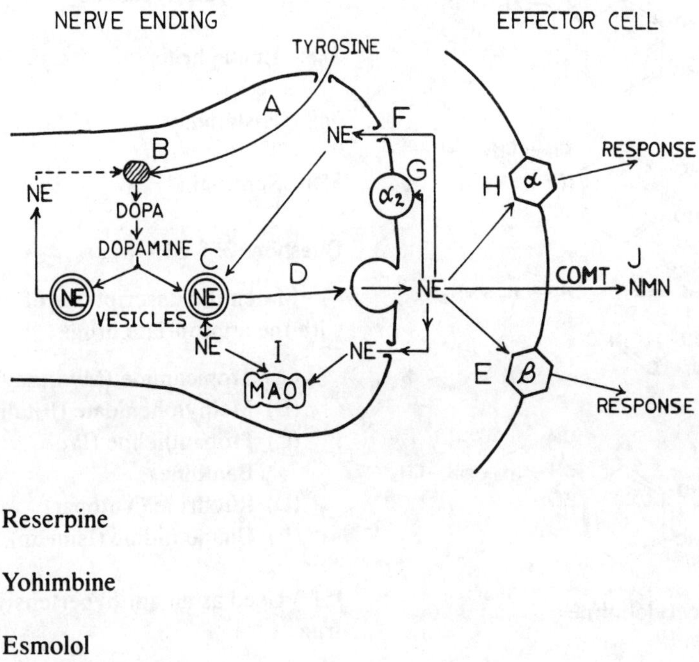

341. Reserpine

342. Yohimbine

343. Esmolol

344. Tranylcypromine

Questions 345–347

For each of the naturally occurring amines below, select the appropriate structure.

A 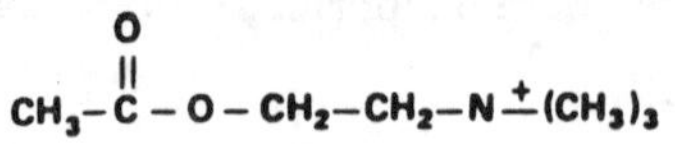

B 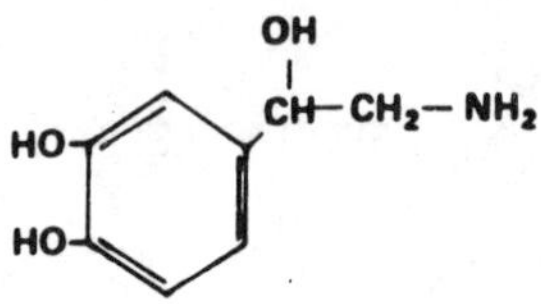

C 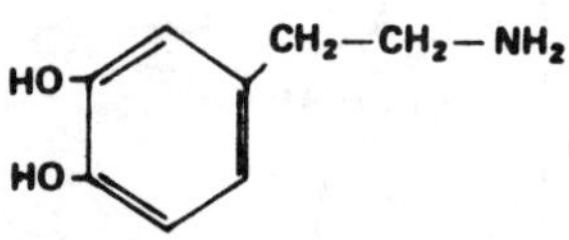

D 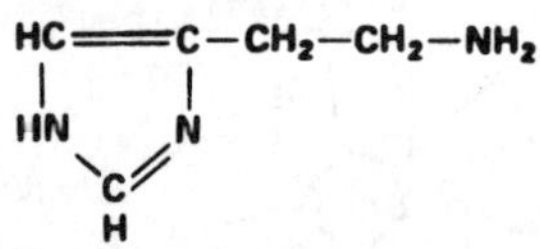

E 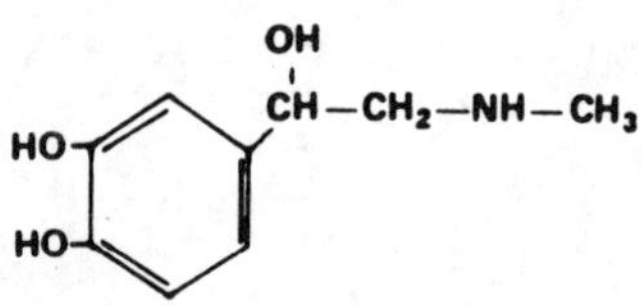

345. Acetylcholine

346. Histamine

347. Epinephrine

Questions 348–350

For each of the neurotransmitters below, select the amino acid from which it is synthesized.

(A) Tyrosine
(B) Serine
(C) Histidine
(D) Tryptophan
(E) Hydroxyproline

348. Epinephrine

349. Histamine

350. Serotonin

Questions 351–353

Match the descriptions of use with the appropriate drug.

(A) Tropicamide (Mydriacyl)
(B) Methylphenidate (Ritalin)
(C) Propantheline (Pro-Banthine)
(D) Ritodrine (Yutopar)
(E) Guanethidine (Ismelin)

351. Used as an antihypertensive drug

352. Used in the treatment of gastrointestinal hypermotility

353. Used as an adjunct in the therapy of hyperkinetic syndromes

Questions 354–359

For each of the drugs below, select its appropriate site of action in the acetylcholine system diagrammed.

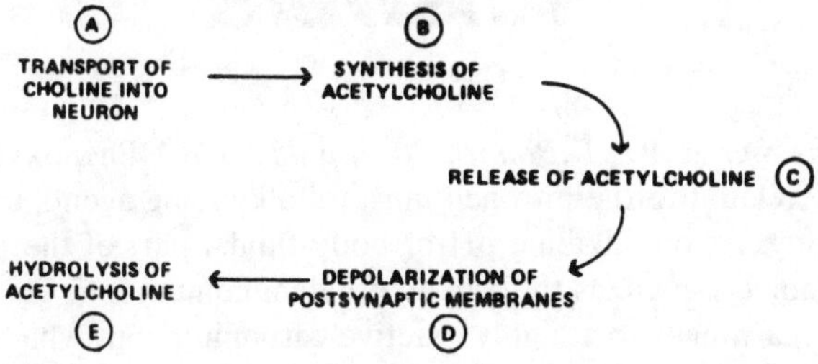

354. Botulinus toxin

355. Isoflurophate

356. Tubocurarine

357. Hemicholinium

358. Hexamethonium

359. Muscarine

Autonomic Nervous System

Answers

290. The answer is B. *(DiPalma, 3/e. pp 119–123.)* Phenoxybenzamine is structurally related to the nitrogen mustard alkylating agents used in cancer chemotherapy. At the alkaline pH of body fluids, part of the molecule (the N—C—C moiety) cyclizes to form an ethylenimonium ion. This unstable intermediate rearranges to a highly reactive carbonium ion, which forms a stable covalent bond with $alpha_1$- and $alpha_2$-adrenoceptors.

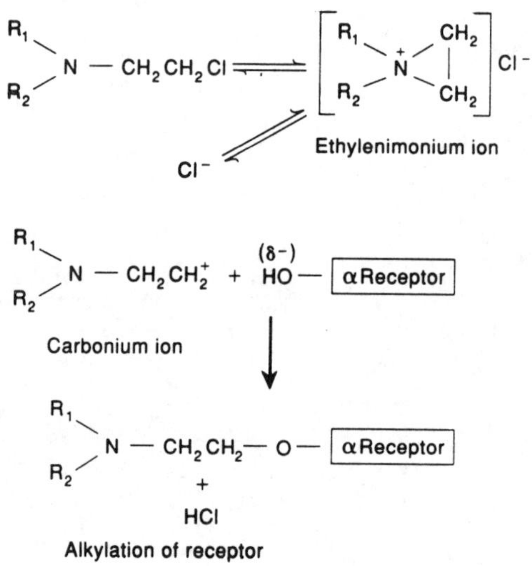

This long-lasting receptor blockade cannot be overcome by competition with an agonist. Therefore, in contrast to phentolamine, prazosin, terazosin, and ergotamine (all reversible *competitive* alpha-adrenergic receptor antagonists), blockade with phenoxybenzamine is not reversible and is referred to as *nonequilibrium receptor blockade*.

291. The answer is D. *(DiPalma, 3/e. pp 132–133. Gilman, 8/e. pp 180–181.)* Nicotine is a depolarizing ganglionic blocking agent; that is, it stimulates nicotinic receptors in low doses and predominantly blocks at high dose levels. The effect of nicotine on a particular tissue or organ depends on the relative contribution to function made by each division of the autonomic nervous system. The effects on the cardiovascular system are complex. Stimulation of the cardiac vagal ganglia causes bradycardia. This is countered by sympathetic stimulation to the heart (tachycardia), blood vessels (vasoconstriction), and adrenal medulla (catecholamine release: tachycardia and vasoconstriction). Thus the net effect of nicotine on the heart is tachycardia, not bradycardia. Low doses of nicotine augment respiration by excitation of the chemoreceptors of the carotid body and aortic arch. Higher doses also stimulate the medullary respiratory center and increase respiration through CNS activity. Large amounts of nicotine cause respiratory failure from medullary paralysis and blockade of the skeletal muscles of respiration.

292. The answer is B. *(DiPalma, 3/e. pp 139, 167, 170, 174, 256.)* Many compounds from diverse pharmacologic categories elicit antimuscarinic (anticholinergic) effects. As an example, diphenhydramine (an antihistamine), meperidine (an opioid analgesic), amitriptyline (an antidepressant), and thioridazine (an antipsychotic) all produce clinically significant antimuscarinic effects. In some cases, these become annoying adverse reactions, e.g., dryness of the mouth and tachycardia, as seen with amitriptyline. In other instances this property can be useful; e.g., reduced nasal secretions enhance the utility of diphenhydramine in the therapy of colds and allergies.

Pyridostigmine does not have antimuscarinic activity; rather, it *produces* muscarinic and nicotinic effects. This drug is an indirect-acting cholinomimetic agent that inhibits the activity of acetylcholinesterase and plasma cholinesterase, the enzymes that hydrolyze acetylcholine. Pyridostigmine is used as the drug of choice for oral therapy of myasthenia gravis.

293. The answer is B. *(DiPalma, 3/e. p 100.)* Endogenous catecholamines such as epinephrine and norepinephrine are rather labile in the body; they are readily biotransformed to inactive products by digestive secretions and enzymes of the intestinal mucosa and liver. Owing to their low lipid-to-water partition coefficients, these drugs penetrate biologic membranes poorly, and molecules that are absorbed cause vasoconstriction of the portal circulation, which further reduces the oral bioavailability of these drugs. The parenteral administration of epinephrine is usually by subcutaneous or intramuscular injection. Norepinephrine, although rarely used, is always administered intravenously. Some drugs, e.g., the tetracycline antibiotics, will complex with divalent cations (aluminum, calcium, iron) in the gastrointestinal tract and their oral absorption will be inhibited; this does not occur with epinephrine and norepinephrine.

294. The answer is B. *(AMA Drug Evaluations Annual 1991, 7/e. pp 1820–1821. DiPalma, 3/e. pp 134, 136, 140–142.)* Echothiophate iodide is a long-acting (irreversible) cholinesterase inhibitor. It is used topically in the eye for the treatment of various types of glaucoma. Maximum reduction of intraocular pressure occurs within 24 h and the effect may persist for several days. The drug is a water-soluble compound, which affords it a practical advantage over the lipid-soluble isoflurophate (another cholinesterase inhibitor used to treat glaucoma).

295. The answer is D. *(DiPalma, 3/e. pp 148–149. Gilman, 8/e. pp 157–158.)* The history and clinical findings in the patient presented in the question are indicative of widespread parasympathetic blockade. Symptoms and signs of such blockade should immediately arouse suspicion of atropine poisoning or intoxication by another drug with significant anticholinergic activity. When atropine poisoning is suspected but questionable, subcutaneous injection of 1 mg of physostigmine (Antilirium) can be diagnostic; if salivation, sweating, and intestinal hyperactivity do not occur following the injection, anticholinergic intoxication is almost certain.

296. The answer is D. *(DiPalma, 3/e. pp 94–98, 358, 440. Gilman, 8/e. pp 201–202.)* Isoproterenol is a nonselective beta-adrenergic receptor agonist. Cardiac stimulation (via $beta_1$-receptors), relaxed bronchial smooth muscle, and vasodilation (via $beta_2$-receptors) are typical effects observed following the administration of the drug. Based on these effects, isoproterenol is used as a cardiac stimulant in heart block and shock (by injection) and as a bronchodilator in respiratory disorders (by inhalation). The drug is short-acting since it is metabolized primarily and efficiently by catechol-*O*-methyltransferase (COMT). It is a relatively poor substrate for MAO, however.

297. The answer is E. *(DiPalma, 3/e. p 118. Gilman, 8/e. pp 235–236.)* With the exception of acebutolol—which is classified as a "cardioselective," or selective, $beta_1$-adrenergic blocking agent—all the listed drugs are considered to be nonselective beta-adrenergic blocking agents because they will competitively antagonize agonists at both $beta_1$- and $beta_2$-adrenergic receptor sites. Labetalol is unique in that it is, at therapeutic doses, also a competitive antagonist at $alpha_1$-adrenergic receptors. The drug has more potent blocking activity at beta-adrenoceptors; the potency ratio for alpha:beta blockade is 1:3 for the oral route and 1:7 after intravenous administration. Similar to the other beta-adrenergic blocking drugs, labetalol is indicated for the treatment of essential hypertension; however, because of the $alpha_1$-adrenergic blocking activity, blood pressure is often decreased more in the standing than in the supine position and symptoms of postural hypotension can occur.

298. The answer is A. *(Katzung, 4/e. pp 209–210.)* The enterochromaffin cells of the intestine contain about 90 percent of the mammalian body's serotonin, known chemically as 5-hydroxytryptamine (5-HT). This endogenous amine causes gastrointestinal smooth muscle to contract by both a direct action on 5-HT receptors of the muscle and by stimulation of parasympathetic ganglia found within the intestinal wall. Although it is believed that serotonin serves a physiologic function by increasing tone and facilitating peristalsis, it may also be involved in certain diseases, e.g., carcinoid tumor, in which an overproduction of serotonin results in diarrhea.

299. The answer is E. *(DiPalma, 3/e. p 116. Gilman, 8/e. pp 238–239.)* Propranolol is a competitive antagonist of both $beta_1$- and $beta_2$-adrenergic receptors. Since the sympathetic division of the autonomic nervous system may be a vital component in support of cardiac performance in many patients with congestive heart failure, $beta_1$-adrenergic blockade may precipitate more severe depression of cardiac function. The $beta_2$-adrenoceptors in the bronchioles of patients with bronchospastic disease (e.g., bronchial asthma, chronic bronchitis, emphysema) are important in mediating bronchodilation; thus, blockade of these receptors may cause a severe increase in airway resistance, thereby decreasing pulmonary function in such patients, which may be life-threatening. Propranolol should also be used with caution in diabetic patients who are prone to hypoglycemia since beta-adrenergic blockers may mask the warning signs of acute hypoglycemia (e.g., tachycardia). Some patients who use propranolol and other beta-adrenergic blockers complain of cold extremities. Since these drugs may mildly elevate peripheral resistance, they should be used with caution in patients with vasospastic diseases such as Raynaud's phenomenon and acrocyanosis. There is no contraindication or warning concerning the use of propranolol in angina pectoris; rather, propranolol and other beta-adrenergic blocking agents are indicated for the treatment of this disease. There have been reports, however, of exacerbation of angina following abrupt discontinuation of these drugs.

300. The answer is B. *(DiPalma, 3/e. p 82. Gilman, 8/e. pp 89–90.)* The radial muscle of the iris contains predominantly alpha-adrenergic receptors; when exposed to such alpha-receptor agonists as phenylephrine, the muscle contracts, resulting in mydriasis. Miosis occurs when the ciliary muscle, which contains beta-receptors, relaxes. Bronchial muscle, the atrioventricular node, and the sinoatrial node are among other sites that contain beta-receptors and respond to beta-adrenergic agonists.

301. The answer is C. *(DiPalma, 3/e. pp 111, 124–126. Gilman, 8/e. pp 475, 794–796.)* Selegiline (also known as *deprenyl*) is a selective monoamine oxidase (MAO) inhibitor that is used to treat Parkinson's disease. At recommended doses, the drug inhibits MAO type B (found mainly in the brain), with little effect on MAO type A (found predominantly in the intestine and liver). Inhibition of MAO will tend to raise the pool of catecholamine neurotransmitters (norepinephrine, dopamine) available for release by sympathetic neurons.

Guanadrel and guanethidine are adrenergic neuronal blocking drugs that deplete stores of neurotransmitters in sympathetic neurons by competing with catecholamine for binding sites within the storage vesicles. When the sympathetic neurons are depolarized, less neurotransmitter is available to be released. Both of these compounds are used to treat essential hypertension.

Reserpine causes depletion of norepinephrine and dopamine by binding to the membrane of the storage vesicles and irreversibly inhibiting the magnesium-dependent ATP transport process that is responsible for catecholamine uptake into the neuronal vesicles. Like guanethidine and guanadrel, reserpine is indicated for the treatment of essential hypertension.

Metyrosine is a competitive antagonist of tyrosine hydroxylase, the enzyme that converts tyrosine to dihydroxyphenylalanine (DOPA), and the rate-limiting step in the formation of norepinephrine and epinephrine. Metyrosine is used to treat patients with pheochromocytoma, a tumor of the adrenal medulla that produces excessive quantities of these catecholamines and results in hypertension. This compound is not recommended for use in essential hypertension or in hypertension secondary to diseases other than functional adrenal tumors.

302. The answer is E. *(DiPalma, 3/e. pp 105–106. Gilman, 8/e. pp 200–201.)* Dopamine is a mixed-acting sympathomimetic drug that complexes with and activates alpha- and beta$_1$-adrenergic receptors and induces norepinephrine release from sympathetic neurons. Dopamine is unique in that it has little agonistic activity on beta$_2$-adrenergic receptors, but it is a potent stimulant of dopaminergic receptor sites. At low concentrations, activation of D$_1$-dopaminergic receptors in the renal vasculature mediates vasodilation and increased blood flow in this area, resulting in an enhancement of renal function. At somewhat higher concentrations, myocardial beta$_1$-adrenergic receptors are stimulated, resulting in an increased force of contraction; high concentrations of the drug activate vascular alpha-adrenoceptors, which mediate vasoconstriction. Thus dopamine is used for patients with oliguria, with low peripheral resistance, and with some types of shock, e.g., cardiogenic and septic shock. Although dopamine receptors are present in the central nervous system (CNS), the drug does not cross the blood-brain barrier to any significant extent; therefore, CNS adverse reactions are uncommonly observed in most patients. Since dopamine is a catecholamine, it is rapidly inactivated by hepatic monoamine oxidase and catechol-*O*-methyltransferase and, therefore, must be administered by intravenous infusion.

303. The answer is C. *(DiPalma, 3/e. p 159. Gilman, 8/e. p 176.)* Normal plasma cholinesterase enzymatically destroys succinylcholine and is responsible for its short duration of action. Succinylcholine-induced paralysis usually lasts for 5 min (during which time artificial respiration is needed). Patients who are homozygous for a deficient plasma cholinesterase, therefore, remain paralyzed much longer than the average person following the administration of succinylcholine. In rare instances, some people completely lack plasma cholinesterase.

304. The answer is D. *(DiPalma, 3/e. pp 145–146. Gilman, 8/e. pp 154–157.)* Acetylcholine will stimulate both muscarinic and nicotinic receptors. Ganglionic stimulation is an effect of type 1 nicotinic (N1) receptors and skeletal muscle contraction is mediated through N2 receptors. All the other effects listed in the question occur following muscarinic receptor activation and will be blocked by atropine and scopolamine, both of which are muscarinic receptor antagonists. Skeletal muscle contraction will not be affected by these drugs; rather, a neuromuscular blocker (e.g., tubocurarine) is required to antagonize this effect of acetylcholine.

305. The answer is D. *(DiPalma, 3/e. pp 103–104. Gilman, 8/e. pp 205, 632–633.)* Beta-adrenergic receptors are regulatory subunits of adenylate cyclase, the intracellular enzyme that converts adenosine triphosphate (ATP) to cyclic AMP. Selective beta$_2$-adrenergic receptor stimulants (e.g., albuterol, isoetharine, metaproterenol, terbutaline) as well as the nonselective beta-receptor agonists (epinephrine and isoproterenol) all enhance the activity of this enzyme. Like all sympathomimetics, terbutaline and isoetharine elicit CNS side effects, muscle tremors, and, although less than the nonselective beta-receptor agonists, tachycardia. Although the metabolism of each compound is different, extensive first-pass biotransformation of both drugs will occur following oral administration. Isoetharine is a catecholamine, biotransformed by catechol-*O*-methyltransferase (COMT) and is effective only by inhalation. Terbutaline is not biotransformed by COMT, but significant biotransformation via hepatic microsomal enzymes occurs (the oral bioavailability is only about 15 percent). Despite this, oral doses are large enough to compensate and the drug is effective when given orally.

306. The answer is C. *(Gilman, 8/e. pp 234, 239–240.)* In addition to its usefulness in the treatment of hypertension, angina pectoris, supraventricular and ventricular arrhythmias, and in the prophylaxis of migraine headaches, propranolol is indicated for use in hypertrophic subaortic stenosis and pheochromocytoma and to reduce cardiovascular mortality following a myocardial infarction. Propranolol is the beta-adrenergic blocker with the greatest *membrane stabilizing activity* (also known as *local anesthetic activity*). Propranolol applied topically to membranes, such as the cornea, would anesthetize the area; in the case of the eye, this would be detrimental to the patient.

Therefore, this drug is not used for the treatment of glaucoma. Other beta-adrenergic blockers that do not have membrane stabilizing activity—including timolol (Timoptic), betaxolol (Betoptic), and levobunolol (Betagen)—are useful for this purpose. All of these are administered as drops to the eye.

307. The answer is A. *(DiPalma, 3/e. p 102. Gilman, 8/e. p 207.)* Phenylephrine stimulates postsynaptic alpha-adrenergic receptors but has little effect on beta-adrenergic receptors. When applied directly to nasal mucosal tissue, it causes vasoconstriction, which reduces congestion. Phenylephrine is sometimes included in oral preparations, but a dose high enough to be effective as a nasal decongestant would produce generalized vasoconstriction and hypertension.

308. The answer is D. *(DiPalma, 3/e. pp 132–134. Gilman, 8/e. pp 180–181.)* Nicotine is a depolarizing ganglionic blocking agent that initially stimulates and then blocks N1 (ganglionic) and N2 (skeletal muscle) cholinergic receptors. Blockade of the sympathetic division of the autonomic nervous system results in arteriolar vasodilation, bradycardia, and hypotension. Blockade at the neuromuscular junction leads to muscle weakness and respiratory depression caused by interference with the function of the diaphragm and intercostal muscles. Atropine, a muscarinic receptor blocker, would be an effective antagonist, as would neostigmine, a cholinesterase inhibitor. Pilocarpine and isoflurophate are cholinomimetics and can be antagonized by atropine; the effects of tubocurarine can be inhibited by neostigmine. Diazoxide, a vasodilator, would cause tachycardia, rather than bradycardia.

309. The answer is E. *(AMA Drug Evaluations Annual 1991, 7/e. pp 1013–1014.)* Ritodrine hydrochloride is a selective beta$_2$-adrenergic agonist that relaxes uterine smooth muscle. It also has the other effects attributable to beta-adrenergic receptor stimulants, such as bronchodilation, cardiac stimulation, enhanced renin secretion, and hyperglycemia. Of all the selective beta$_2$-adrenergic receptor agonists available in the United States, ritodrine is the only one approved for use in premature labor, although terbutaline sulfate (Brethine) is being evaluated in clinical trials for this indication.

310. The answer is E. *(DiPalma, 3/e. pp 159–160. Katzung, 4/e. pp 332–333.)* There are three major classes of skeletal muscle relaxants: peripherally acting, centrally acting, and direct-acting. The peripherally acting drugs include the nondepolarizing (e.g., tubocurarine, gallamine, pancuronium) and depolarizing (e.g., succinylcholine, decamethonium) neuromuscular blockers that antagonize acetylcholine at the muscle end-plate (i.e., at N2 receptors). Centrally acting skeletal muscle relaxants (e.g., diazepam, cyclobenzaprine, baclofen) interfere with transmission along the monosynaptic and polysynaptic neural pathways in the spinal cord. Dantrolene, the only direct-acting skeletal muscle relaxant, affects the excitation-contraction coupling mechanism of skeletal muscle by depressing the release of ionic calcium from the sarcoplasmic reticulum to the myoplasma. The drug is also useful in the prevention and management of malignant hyperthermia induced by general anesthetics.

311. The answer is C. *(DiPalma, 3/e. p 116. Gilman, 8/e. pp 232–233.)* The chief danger of therapy with beta-adrenergic blocking agents such as nadolol (Corgard) and propranolol (Inderal) is associated with the blockade itself. Beta-adrenergic blockade results in an increase in airway resistance that can be fatal in asthmatic patients. Hypersensitivity reactions such as rash, fever, and purpura are rare and necessitate discontinuation of therapy.

312. The answer is A. *(AMA Drug Evaluations Annual 1991, 7/e. pp 1812, 1815–1816. Gilman, 8/e. pp 143–144, 238, 240.)* When applied topically to the eye, both the direct-acting cholinomimetic agents (e.g., pilocarpine) and those cholinomimetic drugs that act by inhibition of acetylcholinesterase (e.g., echothiophate, isoflurophate, and physostigmine) cause miosis by contracting the sphincter muscle of the iris and reduction of ocular pressure by contraction of the ciliary muscle. In patients with glaucoma, this latter effect permits greater drainage of the aqueous humor through the trabecular meshwork in the canal of Schlemm and a reduction in resistance to outflow of the aqueous humor. Certain beta-adrenergic blocking agents (e.g., betaxolol, timolol, and levobunolol) applied to the eye are also very useful in treating chronic wide-angle glaucoma. These drugs appear to act by decreasing the secretion (or formation) of the aqueous humor by antagonizing the effect of circulating catecholamines on beta-adrenergic receptors in the ciliary epithelium.

313. The answer is D. *(DiPalma, 3/e. pp 130–132, 143. Gilman, 8/e. pp 124, 126–127.)* Of the four choline esters (acetylcholine, methacholine, carbachol, and bethanechol), the latter two drugs have the greatest agonistic activity on muscarinic receptors of the gastrointestinal tract and urinary bladder. Bethanechol is used orally or by subcutaneous injection as a stimulant of the smooth muscles of the gastrointestinal tract (for cases of postoperative abdominal distention, gastric atony and retention or gastroparesis) and the urinary bladder (for nonobstructive postoperative and postpartum urinary retention). Carbachol is not used for these purposes due to significant activity at nicotinic receptors at autonomic ganglia; the drug is useful as a miotic for treating glaucoma and in certain types of ocular surgery. Acetylcholine is occasionally used topically during cataract surgery; metacholine is used by inhalation for the diagnosis of bronchial hyperreactivity in patients who do not have clinically apparent asthma. Pilocarpine (a naturally occurring alkaloid) is a drug of choice for the treatment of glaucoma.

314. The answer is A. *(DiPalma, 3/e. p 139. Gilman, 8/e. p 176.)* Anticholinesterase agents, such as neostigmine, will delay the catabolism of acetylcholine released from parasympathetic autonomic and somatic nerve terminals. At the neuromuscular junction this results in increased competition for the N2 receptors by acetylcholine (the agonist) and the curariform drugs (the antagonists) such as tubocurarine, metocurine, and pancuronium. In addition, neostigmine has a direct stimulating action on the skeletal muscle junction, which enhances its ability to antagonize the competitive neuromuscular blockers. The activity of succinylcholine at the neuromuscular junction will be exacerbated by neostigmine, since succinylcholine is inactivated by acetylcholinesterase. The skeletal muscle relaxation that may result from toxic doses of nicotine-blocking N2 receptors will be unaffected by neostigmine. Diazepam and baclofen are centrally acting skeletal muscle relaxants whose effects are not altered by the peripheral actions of neostigmine.

315. The answer is A. *(DiPalma, 3/e. pp 107–108. Gilman, 8/e. pp 210–213, 217–218.)* Amphetamine and its derivative methamphetamine are sympathomimetic compounds that promote the release of various biogenic amines (e.g., dopamine, norepinephrine, serotonin) from storage vesicles in neurons and are agonists at alpha- and beta-adrenergic receptor sites. Oral administration of amphetamine *raises* both systolic and diastolic blood pressure and may cause heart rate to slow reflexly. The drug is a potent CNS stimulant and evokes excitation, increased alertness, elevation of mood, and insomnia. Anorexia (a loss of appetite) is a common manifestation of amphetamine use and the drug is widely used in the treatment of obesity, although such use is questionable owing to the high potential for abuse of the compound. Amphetamine is approved for use in narcolepsy, a disease characterized by sudden attacks of sleep, and in attention-deficit hyperactivity disorder, a syndrome in children characterized by impulsive behavior, short attention span, and excessive motor activity.

316. The answer is C. *(AMA Drug Evaluations Annual 1991, 7/e. pp 434–438. DiPalma, 3/e. pp 438–442.)* Theophylline, a methylxanthine derivative related to caffeine, is an effective bronchodilator that is used orally in the treatment of chronic obstructive pulmonary diseases, e.g., bronchial asthma. The drug acts by (1) blocking the activity of cyclic nucleotide phosphodiesterase, the enzyme that inactivates cyclic AMP, which allows cyclic AMP to accumulate and cause bronchodilation; and (2) antagonizing adenosine receptors, which, in part, mediate bronchoconstriction. Aminophylline is a more water-soluble salt form of theophylline and has the same actions and effects.

Isoproterenol and albuterol produce relaxation of bronchial smooth muscle by stimulating beta$_2$-adrenergic receptors; albuterol is a selective beta$_2$-adrenergic receptor agonist and isoproterenol stimulates both beta$_1$- and beta$_2$-adrenoceptors. Both of these drugs are commonly used by inhalation; in addition, albuterol is effective following oral administration. Tetrahydrozoline is an alpha-adrenergic receptor agonist that is used for its vasoconstrictor properties as a decongestant. For example, this compound is the active ingredient in Visine (an ocular decongestant) and Tyzine (a nasal decongestant). The drug has little activity on beta-adrenergic receptors and is not an effective bronchodilator.

317. The answer is C. *(DiPalma, 3/e. pp 134–135, 141. Katzung, 4/e. pp 77–78.)* During the hydrolysis of acetylcholine by acetylcholinesterase, the enzyme binds to the substrate by virtue of the electrostatic attraction between the anionic site of the enzyme and the quaternary nitrogen of acetylcholine. In addition, the electrophilic carbon of the carbonyl group of acetylcholine interacts with the nearby nucleophilic esteratic site of the enzyme. As a result of this attraction and interaction, a complex is formed and subsequently cleaved to yield the products choline and the acetylated enzyme. Hydrolysis then rapidly yields acetic acid and the regenerated active enzyme. Those organophosphorus compounds that inhibit cholinesterase activity react with the esteratic site in a manner similar to the processes that occur in the hydrolysis of acetylcholine but phosphorylate rather than acetylate the enzyme. The phosphorylated enzyme does not readily undergo hydrolysis, and thus the enzyme is inactivated.

318. The answer is C. *(DiPalma, 3/e. pp 142–143. Gilman, 8/e. pp 141–142.)* Organophosphate cholinesterase inhibitors react with both acetylcholinesterase and serum cholinesterase (pseudocholinesterase) by phosphorylating the enzymes, thus rendering them inactive, inasmuch as the phosphorylated enzyme hydrolyzes esters very slowly. Pralidoxime chloride (also known as 2-PAM chloride) is an oxime derivative that can cause dephosphorylation of the enzyme if it is administered within a short time after the organophosphate. If not administered promptly, the phosphorylated enzyme will lose an alkyl or alkoxy group (a process called "aging"), leaving a more stable phosphorylated enzyme that then cannot be dephosphorylated. The time period during which this occurs depends upon the nature of the phosphoryl group and the rapidity with which the organophosphate compound affects the enzyme. This can be from a few seconds to several hours.

319. The answer is C. *(Gilman, 8/e. pp 159–160, 162–163, 476.)* A wide variety of clinical conditions are treated with antimuscarinic drugs. Anisotropine methylbromide (Valpin) and methscopolamine bromide (Pamine) have been used to reduce gastrointestinal motility, although side effects—e.g., dryness of the mouth, loss of visual accommodation, and difficulty in urination—usually limit their acceptance by patients. Cyclopentolate hydrochloride (Cyclogyl) is often used in ophthalmology for its mydriatic and cycloplegic properties during refraction of the eye. Trihexyphenidyl hydrochloride (Artane) is one of the important antimuscarinic compounds used in the treatment of parkinsonism. For bronchodilation in patients with bronchial asthma and other bronchospastic diseases, ipratropium bromide (Atrovent) is used by inhalation. Systemic adverse reactions are low since the actions are largely confined to the mouth and airways; additionally, in contrast with atropine, this drug does not affect mucociliary clearance.

320. The answer is D. *(DiPalma, 3/e. pp 106–107. Gilman, 8/e. pp 213–214.)* Ephedrine directly stimulates both alpha- and beta-adrenergic receptors and causes release of norepinephrine from adrenergic neurons. Qualitatively its pharmacologic effects resemble those of epinephrine; the drug can increase blood pressure by both vasoconstriction and cardiac stimulation and it will relax bronchiolar smooth muscle. Ephedrine is less potent than epinephrine and the effects observed are usually slower in onset and of longer duration than those of epinephrine. Also in contrast to epinephrine, ephedrine is used orally in many cough and cold preparations for its decongestant activity.

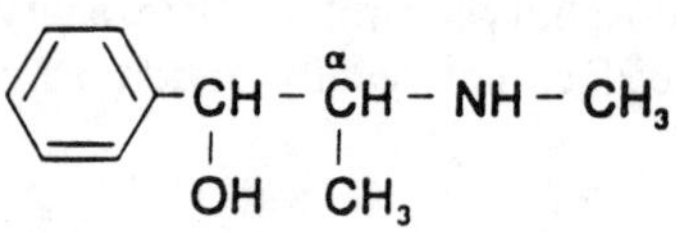

Ephedrine

Ephedrine is quite lipid-soluble compared with epinephrine and will pass through the blood-brain barrier and may cause stimulation of the CNS. Since epinephrine lacks a catechol moiety, it is not biotransformed by COMT and the methyl substitution on the alpha carbon allows the drug to resist oxidation by MAO.

321. The answer is A. *(AMA Drug Evaluations Annual 1991, 7/e. pp 358, 361–362.)* Although all the listed compounds inhibit the activity of the cholinesterases, only edrophonium chloride is used in the diagnosis of myasthenia gravis. The drug has a more rapid onset of action (1 to 3 min following intravenous administration) and a shorter duration of action (approximately 5 to 10 min) than pyridostigmine bromide and ambenonium chloride. It is more water-soluble than physostigmine salicylate and, therefore, produces no clinically significant adverse effects on the CNS. Pyridostigmine bromide and ambenonium chloride are used in the treatment of this muscle weakness disease. Physostigmine salicylate is indicated topically for the treatment of glaucomas and is also a valuable drug for treating toxicity of anticholinergic drugs such as atropine. Malathion is an anticholinesterase that is used topically for the treatment of head lice and is never used internally.

322. The answer is E. *(DiPalma, 3/e. pp 151–152.)* Mecamylamine is a competitive antagonist of acetylcholine at ganglionic cholinergic receptors (N1) and will reduce the activity of both the parasympathetic and the sympathetic divisions of the autonomic nervous system. Since the sympathetic nervous system controls vascular reactivity, mecamylamine will block sympathetic tone to the arterioles, resulting in vasodilation and decreased blood pressure; because of this effect, the drug is used (although rarely today) for the treatment of chronic hypertension. Parasympathetic tone predominates at most other effector structures and, therefore, this drug will affect the heart (tachycardia), eye (mydriasis and cycloplegia), gastrointestinal tract (constipation), urinary bladder (retention of urine), salivary glands (xerostomia), and sweat glands (anhidrosis); these are all adverse manifestations of the compound. Since the nerve pathway to skeletal muscle involves only a single cholinergic motor nerve and no ganglia, and since mecamylamine does not compete with acetylcholine for binding to N2 receptors at the myoneural junction, mecamylamine will have no effect on skeletal muscle tone.

323. The answer is D. *(DiPalma, 3/e. pp 327, 330. Gilman, 8/e. pp 216, 316–317.)* The addition of a vasoconstrictor, such as epinephrine or phenylephrine, to certain short-acting, local anesthetics is a common practice in order to prevent the rapid systemic absorption of the local anesthetic, to prolong the local action, and to decrease the potential systemic reactions. Some local anesthetics cause vasodilation, which allows more compound to escape the tissue and enter the blood. Procaine (Novocaine) is an ester-type local anesthetic with a short duration of action due to rather rapid biotransformation in the plasma by cholinesterases. The duration of action of the drug during infiltration anesthesia is greatly increased by the addition of epinephrine, which reduces the vasodilation caused by procaine.

324. The answer is C. *(DiPalma, 3/e. p 113. Gilman, 8/e. p 234.)* Nonselective beta-adrenergic receptor antagonists block both $beta_1$-receptors (cardiac and renal) and $beta_2$-receptors (bronchial, gastrointestinal, and vascular) and include propranolol, labetalol, nadolol, pindolol, and timolol. Drugs such as acebutolol, atenolol, esmolol, and metoprolol are cardioselective ($beta_1$) adrenergic blocking agents. In either case, the cardiac beta-adrenoceptors are affected by all of these drugs. Haloperidol is a dopamine receptor antagonist; it has no effect on either subtype of beta-adrenergic receptor.

325. The answer is C. *(Gilman, 8/e. p 596. Katzung, 4/e. pp 204–205, 210.)* Cyproheptadine is a potent antihistamine (H_1-receptor antagonist) that has no activity at H_2-receptors. It will block muscarinic receptors and serotonergic receptors. Clinically, it is used for rhinitis, urticaria, and the smooth muscle effects of carcinoid tumor.

326. The answer is B. *(AMA Drug Evaluations Annual 1991, 7/e. pp 592–593. DiPalma, 3/e. p 103.)* At low therapeutic doses, this catecholamine is a selective agonist of myocardial ($beta_1$-adrenergic) receptors; in higher doses, it will lose selectivity and stimulate $beta_2$- and alpha-adrenergic receptor sites. Although it is a structural derivative of dopamine, dobutamine has no activity on peripheral dopaminergic receptors.

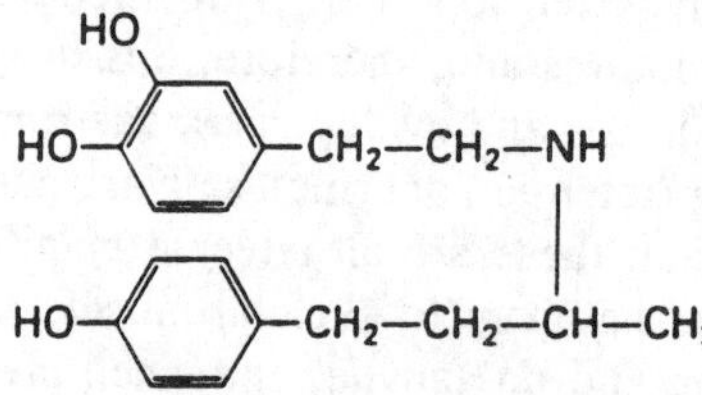

Dobutamine

The drug is not effective orally since it is rapidly biotransformed (plasma $t_{1/2}$ is approximately 2 min) by catechol-*O*-methyltransferase (COMT) and, therefore, must be given by intravenous infusion. It is used to improve myocardial function in patients with severe cardiac failure that has not responded to other treatment modalities. Cardiac adverse effects (e.g., tachycardia and anginal pain) may be observed and represent extensions of the pharmacologic activity of the drug.

327. The answer is D. *(DiPalma, 3/e. p 156. Gilman, 8/e. p 173.)* Flaccid paralysis of all skeletal muscles can be produced by the intravenous administration of large doses of a neuromuscular blocking agent such as tubocurarine. However, not all skeletal musculature is equally sensitive to the action of these drugs. The muscles that produce fine movements—e.g., the extraocular muscles, fingers, and muscles of the head, face, and neck—are most sensitive to these drugs. Muscles of the trunk, abdomen, and extremities are relaxed next, and the respiratory muscles, i.e., the intercostals and the diaphragm, are the most resistant to the action of tubocurarine.

328. The answer is A. *(DiPalma, 3/e. pp 121, 123. Gilman, 8/e. pp 945–946.)* Ergotamine, by virtue of its vasoconstrictive properties rather than its adrenergic blocking action, is the drug of choice for combating an incipient attack of migraine headache. Although chronic treatment with this nonsedative, nonanalgesic drug does not decrease the frequency of or prevent migraine attacks, administration of oral doses is recommended at the beginning of an attack, especially during the prodromal stage. Its use in this setting is recommended despite the fact that ergotamine has a low oral bioavailability due to high first-pass hepatic biotransformation and its effects are much slower after oral administration than when given parenterally. Ergotamine is often combined with caffeine, which enhances the oral absorption of ergotamine. Oral ergotamine provides relief in 5 h and is generally the preferred route for treatment of mild attacks. Administration of this most potent of the ergot alkaloids at the peak of a migraine episode requires effective doses larger than those administered during the prodromal stage and is associated with a delayed onset of action and with a higher incidence of adverse effects, such as nausea, vomiting, pruritus, and disturbances in heart rate.

Propranolol and methysergide are used prophylactically to treat migraine headaches and are not very effective for reducing the pain of migraine headache during an acute attack. Nonopioid analgesics, e.g., aspirin, are not very useful for this type of headache and vasoconstrictors, e.g., pseudoephedrine, are used as nasal decongestants and have no activity on combating migraine headache.

329. The answer is C. *(Gilman, 8/e. pp 88–90.)* Cholinergic impulses arising from the parasympathetic division of the autonomic nervous system affect many tissues and organs throughout the body. Physiologically, this system is concerned primarily with the functions of energy conservation and maintenance of organ function during periods of reduced activity. Slowed heart rate, reduced blood pressure, increased gastrointestinal motility, emptying of the urinary bladder, and stimulation of secretions from the pancreas, salivary glands, lacrimal glands, and bronchial and nasopharyngeal glands are all effects observed due to activation of this nervous system. However, skeletal muscle contraction is mediated through activation of the somatic nervous system, not the autonomic nervous system.

330. The answer is A. *(AMA Drug Evaluations Annual 1991, 7/e. p 1656.)* Epinephrine is the drug of choice to relieve the symptoms of an acute, systemic, immediate hypersensitivity reaction to an allergen (anaphylactic shock). Subcutaneous administration of a 1:1000 solution of epinephrine rapidly relieves itching and urticaria and may save the life of the patient when laryngeal edema and bronchospasm threaten suffocation and severe hypotension and cardiac arrhythmias become life-endangering. Norepinephrine, isoproterenol, and atropine are ineffective therapies. Angioedema is responsive to antihistamines, but epinephrine is necessary in the event of a severe reaction.

331. The answer is A. *(AMA Drug Evaluations Annual 1991, 7/e. pp 507, 509. DiPalma, 3/e. pp 118–120, 123, 428.)* Phentolamine is a nonselective alpha-adrenergic receptor blocker; i.e., it has affinity for both $alpha_1$- and $alpha_2$-adrenergic receptor sites. It also has a prominent direct relaxant (musculotropic spasmolytic) effect on arterioles, which results in vasodilation and reflex tachycardia. In addition, phentolamine can block the effects of serotonin and will increase hydrochloric acid and pepsin secretion from the stomach. Phentolamine is used for the short-term control of hypertension in patients with pheochromocytoma (i.e., a type of secondary hypertension); owing to the high incidence of tachycardia associated with the compound, it is not used chronically for the treatment of primary hypertension.

Prazosin is a selective $alpha_1$-adrenergic receptor antagonist that, at therapeutic doses, has little activity at $alpha_2$-adrenergic receptors and clinically insignificant direct vasodilating activity. The drug does not cause the other effects attributed to phentolamine. Most importantly, it produces less tachycardia than does phentolamine and, therefore, is useful in the treatment of primary hypertension.

332. The answer is C. *(AMA Drug Evaluations Annual 1991, 7/e. p 187. DiPalma, 3/e. p 158.)* Unlike most other neuromuscular blocking agents, cardioacceleration may be observed with both pancuronium bromide and gallamine triethiodide (Flaxedil). The increased heart rate that may be observed with pancuronium appears to be primarily due to an atropine-like antimuscarinic (vagolytic) action on the heart, although other mechanisms have been proposed including (1) release of catecholamines from postganglionic adrenergic cardiac fibers, (2) blockade of neuronal norepinephrine reuptake, and (3) a direct sympathomimetic action. Pancuronium does not cause hypotension, has little ganglionic blocking activity, does not affect the myocardium like digitalis, and does not cross the blood-brain barrier in order to stimulate the vasomotor center.

333. The answer is E. *(Gilman, 8/e. pp 116–118.)* Although acetylcholine and norepinephrine are still considered the major neurotransmitters in the parasympathetic and sympathetic divisions of the autonomic nervous system, respectively, other compounds that exist within autonomic nerve terminals have been found to be released simultaneously during nerve stimulation and are now viewed as cotransmitters or neuromodulators. For example, VIP is localized in a number of parasympathetic neurons, e.g., those that innervate sweat glands and salivary glands, and it appears to function as a cotransmitter with acetylcholine in these structures. ATP and acetylcholine both exist in cholinergic vesicles, and ATP is found within the granules of adrenergic fibers and in the adrenal medulla; this compound is believed to be a neurotransmitter in the gastrointestinal and genitourinary tracts. NPY appears associated with catecholamine-containing neurons and may contribute to vasoconstriction produced by stimulation of the sympathetic nervous system. Although less is known about the function of substance P, this small peptide is found within cholinergic nerves, especially at ganglionic sites, and may function as a neuromodulator. Serotonin (5-hydroxytryptamine) is a neurotransmitter in the CNS; although it may play a role in regulating gastrointestinal motility via peripheral serotonergic neurons, it has not been designated as a cotransmitter or neuromodulator in the autonomic nervous system.

334–337. The answers are: 334-I, 335-C, 336-F, 337-B. *(DiPalma, 3/e. pp 113, 117, 146–147, 153–155. Gilman, 8/e. pp 150–153, 169–174, 226–227, 235.)* Timolol is a beta-adrenergic receptor antagonist. It does not show selectivity for $beta_1$- or $beta_2$-adrenoceptors and, therefore, decreases heart rate by blocking the action of endogenous catecholamines. Timolol, used to lower intraocular pressure in patients with chronic open-angle glaucoma, presumably by decreasing the production of aqueous humor, is more effective than many other types of drugs in the treatment of glaucoma.

Scopolamine is a muscarinic receptor antagonist that easily crosses the blood-brain barrier. The blocking of peripheral muscarinic receptors causes cycloplegia, decreased secretions in the gastrointestinal tract and the lung, urinary retention, and bronchial dilation. Central activity is observed with CNS depression (manifest as drowsiness, amnesia, fatigue) and inhibition of motion sickness.

Atracurium is one of the newer nondepolarizing neuromuscular blocking agents. Similar to tubocurarine, atracurium is a competitive antagonist of acetylcholine at N2 receptors at the myoneural junction of skeletal muscle. At therapeutic doses, these drugs can induce complete paralysis of skeletal muscles, unlike the weaker, centrally acting skeletal muscle relaxants (e.g., diazepam, baclofen, and cyclobenzaprine), which reduce muscular spasms but do not completely block skeletal muscle contractions. The primary therapeutic use of atracurium and other curariform drugs is as an adjunct in surgical anesthesia to relax the skeletal musculature so that surgical manipulations are facilitated.

Doxazosin is a reversible blocker of postsynaptic $alpha_1$-adrenergic receptors, unlike phenoxybenzamine or phentolamine, which are nonselective and react at both presynaptic ($alpha_2$) and postsynaptic ($alpha_1$) receptors. Doxazosin, like its congeners prazosin and terazosin, is used to treat primary hypertension (whereas nonselective alpha-adrenergic antagonists are not) because the drug does not significantly block the negative feedback at presynaptic nerve terminals. When this negative feedback mechanism is blocked by nonselective antagonists, the resulting increase in secretion of the catecholamine neurotransmitter norepinephrine causes a significant increase in heart rate, which is an unacceptable adverse effect in the hypertensive patient.

338–340. The answers are: 338-D, 339-C, 340-A. *(Gilman, 8/e. pp 257–262.)* Dopamine is formed from tyrosine by hydroxylation with tyrosine hydroxylase and the removal of a CO_2 group by aromatic amino acid decarboxylase. The catecholamine is found in high concentrations in parts of the brain: the caudate nucleus, the median eminence, the tuberculum olfactorium, and the nucleus accumbens. Dopamine appears to act as an inhibitory neurotransmitter.

Norepinephrine is synthesized from dopamine by dopamine-β-oxidase, which hydroxylates the β-carbon. This enzyme is localized in the amine storage granules. Norepinephrine is found in adrenergic fibers, the adrenal medulla, and in neurons in the locus ceruleus and lateral ventral tegmental fields of the central nervous system.

Epinephrine is synthesized from norepinephrine in the adrenal medulla. Norepinephrine is methylated by phenylethanolamine-*N*-methyltransferase. Neurons containing this enzyme are also found in the central nervous system.

341–344. The answers are: 341-C, 342-G, 343-E, 344-I. *(DiPalma, 3/e. pp 112–114, 124–125, 274–275. Gilman, 8/e. pp 103, 229, 237, 414–415, 795.)* Reserpine (Serapasil) is an adrenergic neuronal blocking agent that causes depletion of central and peripheral stores of norepinephrine and dopamine. Reserpine acts by irreversibly inhibiting the magnesium-dependent ATP transport process that functions as a carrier for biogenic amines from the cytoplasm of the neuron into the storage vesicle. Depletion of stored norepinephrine results in decreased sympathetic tone; therefore, reserpine causes vasodilation, bradycardia, and hypotension.

Yohimbine (Yohimex) is a competitive antagonist that is selective for $alpha_2$-adrenergic receptors; by blocking these receptors it can attenuate the negative feedback mechanism on the release of norepinephrine. The compound is also an antagonist of serotonin. Yohimbine readily enters the CNS and can increase blood pressure by a central mechanism; it has been used to treat hypotension. The drug is reported to affect erectile function by enhancing norepinephrine release and thus has been used to treat impotence in males, although efficacy has not been clearly demonstrated.

Esmolol hydrochloride (Brevibloc) is a competitive beta-adrenergic receptor antagonist; it is selective for $beta_1$-adrenoceptors. In contrast to pindolol, esmolol has little intrinsic sympathomimetic activity, and it differs from propranolol in that it lacks membrane stabilizing activity. Of all the beta-adrenergic blocking drugs, this compound has the shortest duration of action;

since it is an ester, it is hydrolyzed rapidly by plasma esterases and must be used by the intravenous route. Esmolol is approved only for the treatment of supraventricular arrhythmias.

Tranylcypromine sulfate (Parnate) is an antidepressant drug and an inhibitor of monoamine oxidase (MAO). Its antidepressant effect is probably due to the accumulation of norepinephrine in the brain as a consequence of inhibition of the enzyme. The other two monoamine oxidase inhibitors currently used as antidepressants are isocarboxazid (Marplan) and phenelzine sulfate (Nardil).

345–347. The answers are: 345-A, 346-D, 347-E. *(DiPalma, 3/e. pp 96, 129, 166.)* Acetylcholine, which serves as the neurotransmitter at some synapses within the central nervous system, at autonomic ganglia, and at many peripheral neuroeffector sites, is an ester formed within the cholinergic neuron by the acetylation of choline. The acetylation reaction is catalyzed by the enzyme choline acetyltransferase (choline acetylase). After its release, acetylcholine is usually rapidly hydrolyzed by the enzyme acetylcholinesterase.

Dopamine (C) is the neurotransmitter at selected synapses within the central nervous system and probably within some autonomic ganglia. It is formed within the neuron by the ring hydroxylation of phenylalanine and the subsequent decarboxylation of the resultant dihydroxyphenylalanine. Routes of metabolism of neuronally released dopamine include oxidation by monoamine oxidase and aldehyde dehydrogenase to 3,4-dihydroxyphenylacetic acid and methylation by catechol-*O*-methyltransferase to 3-methoxydopamine.

Norepinephrine (B) is the principal neurotransmitter at peripheral autonomic adrenergic neuroeffector junctions, is synthesized within the adrenergic neuron by the β-hydroxylation of dopamine, and—in contrast to epinephrine—lacks the methyl substituent in the amino group. Much of the neuronally released norepinephrine reenters the adrenergic neuron; reentry into the cell is accomplished by a specific, active transport system.

Histamine is a naturally occurring substance involved in anaphylaxis and allergic reactions. It is formed by the decarboxylation of histidine and is catabolized by two routes: one involving oxidative deamination with subsequent conjugation with ribose, and the other involving ring methylation with subsequent side-chain oxidation.

Epinephrine is a catecholamine released by the adrenal medulla. It is formed by *N*-methylation of norepinephrine, a reaction catalyzed by the enzyme phenylethanolamine-*N*-methyltransferase. In large part, circulating epinephrine is methylated by catechol-*O*-methyltransferase, and the resultant metanephrine undergoes oxidative deamination by monoamine oxidase to yield 3-methoxy-4-hydroxymandelic acid.

348–350. The answers are: 348-A, 349-C, 350-D. *(DiPalma, 3/e. pp 87, 166. Gilman, 8/e. pp 102, 576, 592–593.)* Epinephrine is made from tyrosine in a series of steps through dopa, dopamine, norepinephrine, and finally epinephrine. The conversion of tyrosine to dopa by tyrosine hydroxylase is the rate-limiting step in this pathway. Epinephrine constitutes about 80 percent of the catecholamines in the adrenal medulla. The enzyme that synthesizes epinephrine from norepinephrine is also found in certain areas of the central nervous system.

Histamine, formed by the decarboxylation of histidine, is stored in mast cells and basophils; some other tissues can synthesize histamine but do not store it. Histamine is released from sensitized mast cells during allergic reactions.

Serotonin (5-hydroxytryptamine) is synthesized from tryptophan in two steps. Tryptophan is hydroxylated by tryptophan hydroxylase, and 5-hydroxytryptophan is decarboxylated to give serotonin. Most serotonin in the body is found in the enterochromaffin cells of the intestinal tract and the pineal gland. Platelets take up and store serotonin but do not synthesize it.

351–353. The answers are: 351-E, 352-C, 353-B. *(DiPalma, 3/e. pp 108–109, 126, 149–150, 428. Gilman, 8/e. pp 161–163, 217–218, 794–795.)* Guanethidine inhibits the activity of peripheral sympathetic nerves by impairing neurotransmitter (norepinephrine) release. Chronic administration causes depletion of norepinephrine from intraneuronal storage granules by displacement. Reduced activity of the sympathetic division of the autonomic nervous system leads to bradycardia, vasodilation, and reduced systemic blood pressure.

Propantheline is a semisynthetic antimuscarinic agent, similar to atropine and scopolamine. Its major use is in the treatment of peptic ulcer and gastrointestinal hypermotility. Although less potent than atropine for this purpose, it will produce adverse effects commonly associated with the antimuscarinic group, e.g., xerostomia, tachycardia, and dilated pupils.

Methylphenidate is structurally and pharmacologically related to amphetamine. It is used in both children and adults who are characterized as having attention-deficit disorder (ADD). It has been found to be effective in improving behavior, concentration, and learning ability in 70 to 80 percent of children with ADD. Like amphetamine, it is a CNS stimulant and has significant potential for abuse.

354–359. The answers are: 354-C, 355-E, 356-D, 357-A, 358-D, 359-D. *(DiPalma, 3/e. pp 86, 131–132, 141–142, 151, 153–155.)* Acetylcholine is synthesized from acetyl-CoA and choline. Choline is taken up into the neurons by an active transport system. Hemicholinium blocks this uptake, depleting cellular choline, so that synthesis of acetylcholine no longer occurs.

Botulinus toxin comes from *Clostridium botulinum,* an organism that causes food poisoning. Botulinus toxin prevents the release of acetylcholine from nerve endings by mechanisms that are not clear. Death occurs from respiratory failure caused by the inability of diaphragm muscles to contract.

Tubocurarine is a nondepolarizing agent that binds to the cholinergic receptor at skeletal muscle. It acts as a competitive inhibitor of acetylcholine. Because it is a quaternary ammonium compound, tubocurarine is poorly absorbed from the gastrointestinal tract and is usually given parenterally.

Hexamethonium is also a competitive inhibitor of acetylcholine, but this drug is specific for the nicotinic receptor in the ganglia. Dexamethonium, with 10 carbons instead of 6, is specific for nicotinic receptors at the neuromuscular junction. Hexamethonium causes hypotension by preventing sympathetic constriction of the blood vessels.

Muscarine, an alkaloid from certain species of mushrooms, is a muscarinic receptor agonist. The compound has toxicologic importance; muscarine poisoning will produce all the effects associated with an overdose of acetylcholine, e.g., bronchoconstriction, bradycardia, hypotension, excessive salivary and respiratory secretion, and sweating. Poisoning by muscarine is treated with atropine.

Isoflurophate is an organophosphate inhibitor of acetylcholinesterase that was developed shortly before World War II. Such inhibitors are widely used as insecticides and, on occasion, in the treatment of glaucoma. Isoflurophate reacts irreversibly with acetylcholinesterase so that the action of acetylcholine cannot be terminated.

Renal System

- Carbonic Anhydrase Inhibitors
  - Acetazolamide*
- Loop Diuretics
  - Bumetanide
  - Ethacrynic acid
  - Furosemide*
- Osmotic Diuretics
  - Mannitol
- Potassium-Sparing Diuretics
  - Amiloride
  - Spironolactone*
  - Trimaterene*
- Thiazide Diuretics
  - Bendroflumethiazide
  - Chlorothiazide*
  - Hydrochlorothiazide
  - Polythiazide
- Thiazide-Related Compounds
  - Chlorthalidone
  - Indapamide
  - Metolazone
- Antidiuretic Hormone
  - Vasopressin*
  - Desmopressin
  - Lypressin

DIRECTIONS: Each question below contains five suggested responses. Select the **one best** response to each question.

360. The structure shown below is a member of which of the following drug groups?

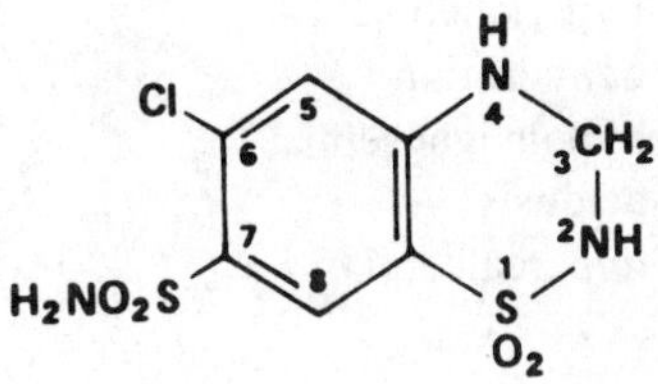

(A) Osmotic diuretics
(B) Loop diuretics
(C) Thiazide diuretics
(D) Potassium-sparing diuretics
(E) Carbonic anhydrase inhibitors

361. The synergistic effect from the combined use of a loop diuretic and a thiazide is due to reduction of sodium chloride reabsorption in the

(A) collecting duct
(B) ascending limb of the loop of Henle
(C) descending limb of the loop of Henle
(D) proximal tubule
(E) distal convoluted tubule

362. Canrenone, which elicits a diuretic response, is a major biotransformation product of which of the following agents?

(A) Indapamide (Lozol)
(B) Chlorthalidone (Hygroton)
(C) Spironolactone (Aldactone)
(D) Amiloride (Midamor)
(E) Triamterene (Dyrenium)

363. Mannitol may be useful in all the following procedures EXCEPT

(A) treatment of elevated intracranial pressure
(B) treatment of elevated intraocular pressure
(C) treatment of pulmonary edema with congestive heart failure
(D) diagnostic evaluation of acute oliguria
(E) prophylaxis of acute renal failure

364. True statements about triamterene (Dyrenium) include all the following EXCEPT

(A) it has a shorter duration of action than spironolactone
(B) it is a weak diuretic
(C) it is used with hydrochlorothiazide in treating hypertension
(D) it is biotransformed by hydroxylation and conjugation
(E) it can produce hyperglycemia

365. Adverse interactions may occur between thiazides and all the following drug groups EXCEPT

(A) adrenal corticosteroids
(B) anticoagulants (oral)
(C) aminoglycosides
(D) beta-adrenergic blockers
(E) antidepolarizing skeletal muscle relaxants

366. Hyperkalemia is a contraindication to the use of which of the following drugs?

(A) Acetazolamide (Diamox)
(B) Chlorothiazide (Diuril)
(C) Ethacrynic acid (Edecrin)
(D) Chlorthalidone (Hygroton)
(E) Spironolactone (Aldactone)

367. A reduction in insulin release from the pancreas may be caused by which of the following diuretics?

(A) Triamterene (Dyrenium)
(B) Chlorothiazide (Diuril)
(C) Spironolactone (Aldactone)
(D) Acetazolamide (Diamox)
(E) Amiloride (Midamor)

368. Acute uric acid nephropathy, which is characterized by the acute overproduction of uric acid and by extreme hyperuricemia, can best be prevented with

(A) antidiuretic hormone (vasopressin, ADH)
(B) cyclophosphamide (Cytoxan)
(C) allopurinol (Zyloprim)
(D) amiloride (Midamor)
(E) sodium chloride

369. Idiopathic calcium urolithiasis can be treated by the administration of

(A) ethacrynic acid (Edecrin)
(B) triamterene (Dyrenium)
(C) furosemide (Lasix)
(D) hydrochlorothiazide (Hydrodiuril)
(E) bumetanide (Bumex)

370. A hospitalized patient, who has been maintained on parenteral alimentation for 3 weeks, develops weakness, tremors, agitation, and finally coma. The most likely fluid and electrolyte disturbance is

(A) hyperkalemia
(B) dehydration
(C) hypomagnesemia
(D) acidosis
(E) hypercalcemia

371. The release of antidiuretic hormone (ADH) is suppressed by which of the following drugs to promote a diuresis?

(A) Guanethidine (Ismelin)
(B) Acetazolamide (Diamox)
(C) Chlorothiazide (Diuril)
(D) Ethanol
(E) Indomethacin (Indocin)

375. Adverse reactions reported with administration of chlorthalidone (Hygroton) include all the following EXCEPT

(A) hyperlipidemia
(B) hyponatremia
(C) hypokalemia
(D) hyperuricemia
(E) hyperglycemia

373. Antidiuretic hormone (vasopressin) is used therapeutically for

(A) increasing uterine contractility
(B) treating nephrogenic diabetes insipidus
(C) treating pituitary diabetes insipidus
(D) treating polyuria caused by hypercalcemia
(E) decreasing chest pain in refractory unstable angina

374. Properties of mannitol include all the following EXCEPT

(A) retention of water in the tubular fluid
(B) the ability to be metabolically altered to an active form
(C) the capacity to be freely filtered
(D) effectiveness as nonelectrolytic, osmotically active particles
(E) the ability to resist complete reabsorption by the renal tubule

375. True statements about indapamide (Lozol) include all the following EXCEPT

(A) it is extensively biotransformed
(B) it is well absorbed orally
(C) it is used in the treatment of hypertension
(D) it inhibits sodium and chloride reabsorption in the distal tubule of the nephron
(E) duration of action is about 4 to 6 h

376. Conservation of potassium ions in the body occurs with which of the following diuretics?

(A) Furosemide (Lasix)
(B) Hydrochlorothiazide (Hydrodiuril)
(C) Amiloride (Midamor)
(D) Metolazone (Zaroxolyn)
(E) Bumetanide (Bumex)

377. Spironolactone (Aldactone) can be characterized by which one of the following statements?

(A) It is biotransformed to an inactive product
(B) It binds to a cytoplasmic receptor
(C) It is a more potent diuretic than is hydrochlorothiazide
(D) It interferes with aldosterone synthesis
(E) It inhibits sodium reabsorption in the proximal renal tubule of the nephron

378. Adverse reactions associated with furosemide (Lasix) include all the following EXCEPT

(A) hyperglycemia
(B) tinnitus
(C) fluid and electrolyte imbalance
(D) hypertension
(E) metabolic acidosis

379. The distal tubule of the nephron is the principal site of action for which one of the following?

(A) Bumetanide (Bumex)
(B) Hydrochlorothiazide (Hydrodiuril)
(C) Ethacrynic acid (Edecrin)
(D) Triamterene (Dyrenium)
(E) Amiloride (Midamor)

380. Chlorothiazide increases the urinary excretion of all the following ions EXCEPT

(A) potassium
(B) chloride
(C) calcium
(D) sodium
(E) magnesium

381. The increased urinary excretion of sodium, potassium, magnesium, and calcium occurs with the administration of

(A) spironolactone (Aldactone)
(B) chlorothiazide (Diuril)
(C) ethacrynic acid (Edecrin)
(D) acetazolamide (Diamox)
(E) amiloride (Midamor)

382. Adverse reactions associated with both acetazolamide (Diamox) and antibacterial sulfonamides include all the following EXCEPT

(A) formation of urinary calculi
(B) fever
(C) metabolic acidosis
(D) crystalluria
(E) exfoliative dermatitis

383. Hydrochlorothiazide is clinically useful in the treatment of all the following EXCEPT

(A) edema caused by congestive heart failure
(B) edema induced by glucocorticoids
(C) hypertension with or without edema
(D) liver disease with ascites
(E) glaucoma by reduction of intraocular pressure

384. Which of the following agents causes a reduction in the hypertonicity of the medullary interstitium of the kidney?

(A) Metolazone (Zaroxolyn)
(B) Spironolactone (Aldactone)
(C) Hydrochlorothiazide (Hydrodiuril)
(D) Mannitol
(E) Ethacrynic acid (Edecrin)

385. An enhancement of the parathyroid hormone–mediated reabsorption of calcium in the distal tubule is caused by which of the following diuretics?

(A) Acetazolamide (Diamox)
(B) Furosemide (Lasix)
(C) Triamterene (Dyrenium)
(D) Bumetanide (Bumex)
(E) Hydrochlorothiazide

DIRECTIONS: Each group of questions below consists of lettered headings followed by a set of numbered items. For each numbered item select the **one** lettered heading with which it is **most** closely associated. Each lettered heading may be used **once, more than once, or not at all.**

Questions 386–389

For each of the diuretic agents below, choose the anatomic site in the renal nephron where the principal action of the agent occurs.

(A) Glomerulus
(B) Proximal tubule
(C) Ascending limb of the loop of Henle
(D) Distal tubule
(E) Collecting duct

386. Acetazolamide (Diamox)

387. Amiloride (Midamor)

388. Bumetanide (Bumex)

389. Metolazone (Zaroxolyn)

Questions 390–391

For each clinical application below, select the most appropriate group of agents.

(A) Osmotic diuretics
(B) High-ceiling, or loop, diuretics
(C) Thiazide (benzothiadiazide) diuretics
(D) Carbonic anhydrase inhibitors
(E) Aldosterone antagonists

390. Treatment of glaucoma

391. Very rapid and brief diuresis

Questions 392–394

Match each statement with the appropriate drug.

(A) Metolazone
(B) Ethacrynic acid
(C) Chlorthalidone
(D) Triamterene
(E) Spironolactone
(F) Acetazolamide
(G) Furosemide
(H) Mannitol
(I) Amiloride
(J) Hydrochlorothiazide

392. The urinary excretion of chloride is decreased

393. Elevated intraocular and cerebrospinal fluid pressures are reduced

394. Chemically, this compound is a steroid

Renal System

Answers

360. The answer is C. *(DiPalma, 3/e. pp 410–411, 415. Gilman, 8/e. p 720.)* The structure shown in the question is hydrochlorothiazide (Esidrix) and is one of several of the thiazide (benzothiadiazide) diuretics. Halogenation of the benzothiadiazine ring at C 6 and a free sulfamyl group (—SO_2NH_2) at C 7 are necessary for maximal diuretic activity in the series of compounds. In contrast to the carbonic anhydrase inhibitors, benzothiadiazides can act independently of acid-base balance. An example of an osmotic diuretic is mannitol; representatives of the loop diuretics are furosemide, ethacrynic acid, and bumetanide. Potassium-sparing diuretics are spironolactone (a steroid), triamterene (a pyrazine derivative), and amiloride (a pyrazinecarbonylguanidine).

361. The answer is D. *(DiPalma, 3/e. pp 412, 415. Katzung, 4/e. pp 184, 191.)* In the treatment of edema some patients become refractory to the loop or high-ceiling diuretic, such as furosemide. It is reported that these patients respond to the combination of a loop diuretic and a thiazide compound. The site of action for this synergistic effect appears to be the proximal tubule. The thiazide alone can inhibit proximal tubular reabsorption of sodium chloride; however, the sodium chloride is readily taken up by the ascending limb of the loop of Henle. The diuretic effect of the thiazide that is administered by itself is actually due to the blockade of sodium chloride reabsorption in the distal convoluted tubule. Thus, when a thiazide and a loop diuretic are used together, the overall result is to enhance the sodium excretion in the proximal tubule. The final result is a profound diuresis. The addition of a thiazide diuretic to a loop diuretic also lessens the incidence of adverse reactions that might occur if only higher doses of the loop diuretic are used to decrease the edema in the patient.

362. The answer is C. *(DiPalma, 3/e. pp 415–416. Gilman, 8/e. pp 725–728.)* Canrenone is the active biotransformation product of spironolactone. Similar to spironolactone, it is a competitive antagonist of aldosterone in the collecting duct of the nephron. Canrenone, like spironolactone, can bind to the cytoplasmic aldosterone receptor and prevent the receptor from being converted to the active conformation. Since the active conformation is prevented, reduction of sodium chloride reabsorption and potassium retention results. The diuretic action of spironolactone is partially due to the presence of canrenone. Indapamide, chlorthalidone, amiloride, and furosemide are not biotransformed to active products. Triamterene, however, is converted to some products that exhibit diuretic activity.

363. The answer is C. *(DiPalma, 3/e. p 418. Gilman, 8/e. pp 714–715.)* Mannitol increases serum osmolarity and therefore "pulls" water out of cells, cerebrospinal fluid, and aqueous humor. This effect can be useful in the treatment of elevated intraocular or intracranial pressure. However, by expanding the intravascular volume, mannitol can exacerbate congestive heart failure. Mannitol will increase urine output if oliguria is caused by a decreased glomerular filtration rate but not if the oliguria is secondary to tubular dysfunction. Mannitol is useful in the prevention of acute renal failure as a means of maintaining an adequate flow of relatively dilute urine.

364. The answer is E. *(DiPalma, 3/e. pp 412, 414, 416–417. Katzung, 4/e. p 192.)* Triamterene is a potassium-sparing diuretic that possesses a weak diuretic effect and can be combined with hydrochlorothiazide to prevent the development of hypokalemia in the therapy of edema and hypertension. The compound is extensively biotransformed in the liver by hydroxylation and conjugation and has a shorter duration of action (12 to 16 h) than spironolactone (48 to 72 h), which is less extensively biotransformed. Hyperglycemia is associated with thiazide and loop diuretics because they appear to reduce the release of insulin from the pancreas. The potassium-sparing diuretics do not alter the release of insulin.

365. The answer is C. *(AMA Drug Evaluations Annual 1991, 7/e. p 692. DiPalma, 3/e. pp 411–412.)* Drug interactions are reported for various drugs and the thiazide diuretics. Thiazides can indirectly promote the loss of potassium from the collecting duct of the nephron, and adrenal corticosteroids can enhance the hypokalemic effect. The therapeutic effect of oral anticoagulants may be reduced by thiazides because these diuretics can concentrate clotting factors in the blood. Thiazide diuretics elevate blood lipid, urate, and glucose levels and these effects can be augmented in the presence of a beta-adrenergic blocker. In addition, the neuromuscular blocking action of tubocurarine is enhanced by thiazide diuretics. Aminoglycosides, which can cause eighth nerve damage, can increase the ototoxicity that is associated with the use of the loop diuretics. Tinnitus and ototoxicity have not been reported as adverse reactions for the thiazide diuretics.

366. The answer is E. *(DiPalma, 3/e. pp 415–416. Gilman, 8/e. p 726.)* Spironolactone (Aldactone) is a competitive antagonist of aldosterone that blocks the reabsorption of sodium and water from the collecting duct in exchange for potassium and hydrogen ion retention. Therefore, in the presence of hyperkalemia, spironolactone is contraindicated. The administration of each of the other diuretic agents listed in the question results in increased excretion of potassium.

367. The answer is B. *(DiPalma, 3/e. pp 412, 414. Gilman, 8/e. p 721.)* An adverse reaction reported to occur occasionally with the thiazides, such as chlorothiazide, is hyperglycemia. In addition hyperglycemia may occur with thiazide-related compounds (chlorothalidone and metolazone) and the high-ceiling diuretics (ethacrynic acid, furosemide, and bumetanide). The proposed mechanism for the elevation in blood glucose appears to be related to a decrease in insulin release from the pancreas. In addition increased glycogenolysis, decreased glycogenesis, and a reduction in the conversion of proinsulin to insulin may also be involved in the hyperglycemic response. Diazoxide, a nondiuretic thiazide, is given to treat hypoglycemia in certain conditions. However, diazoxide is used more often to control hypertensive emergencies.

368. The answer is C. *(DiPalma, 3/e. pp 342, 647. Gilman, 8/e. p 678.)* Acute hyperuricemia, which often occurs in patients treated with cytotoxic drugs for neoplasic disorders, can lead to the deposition of urate crystals in the kidneys and their collecting ducts. This can produce partial or complete obstruction of the collecting ducts, renal pelvis, or ureter. Allopurinol and its primary metabolite, alloxanthine, are inhibitors of xanthine oxidase, an enzyme that catalyzes the oxidation of hypoxanthine and xanthine to uric acid. The use of allopurinol in patients at risk can markedly reduce the likelihood that they will develop acute uric acid nephropathy.

369. The answer is D. *(DiPalma, 3/e. pp 410, 413, 415. Katzung, 4/e. pp 118, 190.)* In the nephron unit calcium ions are reabsorbed from the renal tubular fluid in the cortical portion of the ascending limb of Henle and in the distal tubule. Parathyroid hormone mediates the transport of calcium in the distal tubule. Thiazide diuretics and thiazide-related compounds enhance the reabsorption of calcium ions in the distal tubule and therefore reduce urinary excretion of calcium. This effect of thiazide diuretics and related compounds makes these drugs useful in the treatment of idiopathic calcium urolithiasis. The loop diuretics such as furosemide, bumetanide, and ethacrynic acid tend to enhance the urinary excretion of calcium. They reduce the reabsorption of calcium in the ascending limb of the loop of Henle and, therefore, lower serum levels of calcium. These drugs are effective in the acute treatment of hypercalcemia.

370. The answer is C. *(Gilman, 8/e. p 705.)* Hypomagnesemia is characterized by signs and symptoms that usually include disturbances in the nervous and muscular systems, psychotic behavior, tetany, tachycardia, and hypertension. Because few parenteral alimentation fluids contain magnesium, the clinical manifestations of hypomagnesemia are most commonly found in association with the prolonged parenteral alimentation of magnesium-free solutions.

371. The answer is D. *(DiPalma, 3/e. pp 235, 410, 417. Gilman, 8/e. p 374.)* Ethanol produces a diuretic response by inhibiting the release of antidiuretic hormone (ADH) from the posterior pituitary gland. Less antidiuretic hormone acts on the collecting duct of the nephron and, therefore, the amount of water reabsorbed by the collecting duct is reduced. Indomethacin enhances the release of antidiuretic hormone, which increases the permeability of the collecting duct to water. Acetazolamide and chlorothiazide promote a diuresis by acting on site directly in the nephron unit to reduce the reabsorption of sodium chloride and water. Guanethidine, an antihypertensive agent, does not appear to alter the release of antidiuretic hormone.

372. The answer is A. *(DiPalma, 3/e. pp 412–413. Gilman, 8/e. pp 718–721.)* Adverse reactions reported with the administration of thiazide-like diuretics such as chlorthalidone include hypokalemia and hyperuricemia. In the nephron unit of the kidney, thiazide-like agents cause an increased excretion of sodium and chloride ions and the loss of potassium ions. Chlorthalidone may also produce a loss of bicarbonate ion since it possesses some carbonic anhydrase inhibitory activity. The hypokalemia may be treated with the administration of potassium chloride or by the administration of a potassium-sparing diuretic such as spironolactone, triamterene, or amiloride. Hyperuricemia may be produced by the competition of the diuretic with the secretory pathway for uric acid. Although chlorthalidone occasionally may induce hyperglycemia, it can be used in patients with diabetes mellitus if the patient is carefully evaluated and followed by the physician. Unlike the thiazide diuretics (e.g., hydrochlorothiazide), chlorthalidone does not cause hyperlipidemia.

373. The answer is C. *(Katzung, 4/e. pp 462–463.)* Small doses of antidiuretic hormone (vasopressin) or the newer synthetic analogue, desmopressin, can control polyuria and polydipsia in diabetes insipidus caused by pituitary insufficiency. Other syndromes that mimic the polyuria of vasopressin deficiency, such as nephrogenic diabetes insipidus and hypercalcemia, do not respond to antidiuretic hormone (vasopressin). Although antidiuretic hormone (vasopressin) has intrinsic oxytocic activity, it remains relatively ineffective for initiating or intensifying uterine contractions. Antidiuretic hormone is not used in the treatment of angina because the drug produces coronary vasoconstriction. The drug should be used with caution in patients with ischemic heart disease.

374. The answer is B. *(DiPalma, 3/e. pp 418–419. Gilman, 8/e. pp 714–715.)* A significant increase in the amount of any osmotically active solute in voided urine is usually accompanied by an increase in urine volume. Osmotic diuretics effect diuresis through this principle. The osmotic diuretics (such as mannitol) are nonelectrolytes that are freely filtered at the glomerulus, undergo limited reabsorption by the renal tubules, retain water in the renal tubule, and promote an osmotic diuresis, generally without significant sodium excretion. In addition, these diuretics resist alteration by metabolic processes.

375. The answer is E. *(DiPalma, 3/e. pp 412–413. Katzung, 4/e. pp 189–190.)* Indapamide is classified as a diuretic and antihypertensive drug. It is a sulfonamide derivative that has pharmacodynamic properties similar to those of the thiazides. This compound is well absorbed from the gastrointestinal tract (90 percent). Although indapamide undergoes extensive biotransformation in the liver, it has a long duration of action (36 h). The diuresis induced by this drug is due to a reduction in the reabsorption of sodium and chloride ions from the distal tubule of the nephron. Unlike acetazolamide and chlorothiazide, indapamide does not interfere with the catalytic activity of the enzyme carbonic anhydrase. The mechanism for the antihypertensive effect of indapamide is not fully known; however, vasodilation may play a role in the reduction of elevated blood pressure.

376. The answer is C. *(DiPalma, 3/e. pp 411–417. Gilman, 8/e. pp 721–728.)* Amiloride produces retention of the potassium ion by inhibiting in the collecting duct the reabsorption of sodium, which is accompanied by the excretion of potassium ions. The loop diuretics furosemide and bumetanide cause as a possible adverse action the development of hypokalemia. In addition, thiazides (e.g., hydrochlorothiazide) and the thiazide-related agents (e.g., metolazone) can cause the loss of potassium ions with the consequences of hypokalemia. Amiloride is generally given with a loop diuretic or thiazide to prevent or correct the condition of hypokalemia.

377. The answer is B. *(DiPalma, 3/e. pp 415–416. Gilman, 8/e. pp 725–726.)* Spironolactone is a potassium-sparing diuretic. The drug is well absorbed from the gastrointestinal tract and is biotransformed in the liver to an active metabolite, canrenone. Spironolactone is contraindicated in the presence of hyperkalemia, since this aldosterone antagonist may cause further elevation of plasma potassium concentrations. It does not appear to depress adrenal or pituitary function. CNS side effects of the drug can include lethargy, headache, drowsiness, and mental confusion. Spironolactone displaces aldosterone from receptor sites that are responsible for sodium resorption in the collecting duct of the nephron; it does not interfere with the synthesis of aldosterone.

378. The answer is E. *(DiPalma, 3/e. pp 414–415. Gilman, 8/e. pp 723–724.)* The loop, or high-ceiling, diuretics furosemide and ethacrynic acid are cleared by the kidney with such celerity that even high doses repeatedly administered do not result in significant accumulation. Chronic administration of these agents, however, may lead to alkalosis with hyponatremia in association with rapid removal of edema fluid. Other toxic manifestations of loop diuretics include fluid and electrolyte imbalance, gastrointestinal symptoms, interstitial nephritis, hyperglycemia, tinnitus, and infrequent, but serious, ototoxicity. Besides being used as a diuretic agent, furosemide is used in the treatment of hypertension.

379. The answer is B. *(DiPalma, 3/e. pp 410, 412, 413–414, 416–417. Katzung, 4/e. pp 184, 189–192.)* Diuretic agents exert their effect to promote a net loss of sodium and water by blocking the reabsorption of sodium ions at various regions of the nephron unit. The thiazide diuretics (e.g., hydrochlorothiazide) and the thiazide-related compounds (chlorthalidone, metolazone, and indapamide) interfere with the reabsorption of sodium ions in the distal tubule. These diuretics cause an increase in urinary excretion of sodium, chloride, potassium, water, and, in the case of chlorothiazide, bicarbonate. The loop diuretics (e.g., bumetanide, ethacrynic acid, and furosemide) reduce the cotransport of sodium and chloride ions from the ascending limb of the loop of Henle. There occurs an increased urinary excretion of sodium, chloride, potassium, hydrogen, magnesium, and calcium. Since loop diuretics reduce the tonicity of the medullary interstitium, free-water reabsorption is decreased in the collecting duct. The potassium-sparing diuretics (spironolactone, triamterene and amiloride) exert their diuretic action by blocking the reabsorption of sodium in the collecting duct.

380. The answer is C. *(DiPalma, 3/e. pp 410–411. Katzung, 4/e. pp 189–190.)* Thiazide diuretics enhance the excretion of sodium, chloride, potassium, and magnesium ions. The excretion of calcium appears to be reduced following chronic drug administration. Since the thiazide diuretics inhibit sodium chloride reabsorption in the early portion of the distal tubule, an increased load of sodium and chloride ions is presented to the collecting duct. In this region some sodium ions may be actively reabsorbed and potassium ions secreted, which leads to an increased loss of potassium from the body.

381. The answer is C. *(DiPalma, 3/e. pp 410, 413–418. Gilman, 8/e. pp 718–728.)* Ethacrynic acid (Edecrin) produces a rapidity and a degree of diuresis exceeding that caused by other agents. It acts by inhibiting the cotransport of sodium and chloride ions in the ascending portion of Henle's loop and by increasing the rate of flow in the collecting tubules, which promotes the excretion of potassium. Magnesium and calcium ions also are excreted in increased quantities. Thiazide diuretics promote the renal excretion of sodium, chloride, potassium, and magnesium, while they enhance the resorption of calcium ions. Potassium-sparing diuretics (e.g., spironolactone and amiloride) cause the retention of potassium in the blood. The carbonic anhydrase inhibitor acetazolamide increases the excretion of sodium, bicarbonate, and possibly potassium ions.

382. The answer is C. *(DiPalma, 3/e. pp 417–418. Katzung, 4/e. pp 587–589.)* Acetazolamide, an aromatic sulfonamide derivative, is a mild diuretic agent that increases the loss of sodium and water from the body by inhibiting the enzyme carbonic anhydrase. The sulfonamides, a group of antibacterial agents, exert their antimicrobial effect on gram-positive and gram-negative bacteria by competitive antagonism of para-aminobenzoic acid (PABA). Acetazolamide and the sulfonamides are reported to have some similar adverse reactions. Fever, blood dyscrasias, exfoliative dermatitis, skin rash, crystalluria, and formation of calculi may occur with the administration of either. Metabolic acidosis is associated only with the use of acetazolamide. Since this diuretic inhibits carbonic anhydrase in the proximal tubule, plasma levels of bicarbonate decrease, and if the reduction of bicarbonate is significant, metabolic acidosis can develop.

383. The answer is E. *(DiPalma, 3/e. pp 412, 414, 418. Gilman, 8/e. p 721.)* Thiazides are most useful as diuretic agents in the management of edema caused by chronic cardiac decompensation. In the treatment of hypertensive disease, even without obvious edema, thiazides exert a hypotensive action that has proved beneficial. Less common uses of thiazide diuretics include the treatment of edema from glucocorticoids, diabetes insipidus, and hypercalciuria. The carbonic anhydrase inhibitor acetazolamide (Diamox), by inhibiting the secretion of aqueous humor, has the property of decreasing intraocular pressure—an effect of value for patients who have glaucoma. Furosemide is the diuretic agent generally employed to treat acute pulmonary edema, although ethacrynic acid would be effective.

384. The answer is E. *(DiPalma, 3/e. pp 410, 413–414. Katzung, 4/e. pp 184, 187.)* In the ascending limb of the loop of Henle it is the medullary portion of the ascending limb that participates in maintaining the hypertonicity of the interstitium by the cotransport of sodium and chloride from the renal tubular fluid. The medullary hypertonicity contributes to the concentration of urine. The loop diuretics (ethacrynic acid, furosemide, and bumetanide) inhibit the cotransport of sodium and chloride in both the cortical and medullary portions of the ascending limb and reduce the medullary hypertonicity. As a consequence of this action, free-water reabsorption in the collecting duct of the nephron is reduced; therefore, increased amounts of sodium, chloride, and water are excreted from the body.

385. The answer is E. *(DiPalma, 3/e. pp 410, 412. Katzung, 4/e. pp 185, 187, 189–190.)* In the distal tubule of the nephron sodium and chloride ions are reabsorbed. In addition, calcium ions are reabsorbed by a parathyroid-mediated response. Thiazide diuretics (e.g., hydrochlorothiazide) have their site of action on the distal tubule and inhibit the reabsorption of sodium and chloride but enhance the parathyroid-mediated increase of calcium reabsorption. The urinary excretion of sodium and chloride is increased, while excretion of calcium is reduced. Loop diuretics such as furosemide and bumetanide increase the urinary excretion of calcium ions and may be used in the treatment of acute hypercalcemia. Acetazolamide and triamterene do not appear to inhibit the reabsorption of calcium ions in the distal tubule.

386–389. The answers are: 386-B, 387-E, 388-C, 389-D. *(DiPalma, 3/e. pp 410–413, 417–418. Katzung, 4/e. p 184.)* Acetazolamide, a carbonic anhydrase inhibitor, acts mainly in the proximal tubule to reduce the catalytic activity of carbonic anhydrase via cAMP. There results an increased urinary excretion of sodium and bicarbonate and possibly a loss of potassium. Blood acid-base balance, if altered, results in metabolic acidosis.

The newer potassium-sparing diuretic amiloride seems to act to reduce sodium ion reabsorption primarily in the collecting duct. Unlike spironolactone, amiloride is not an aldosterone antagonist. The actual mechanism for amiloride's diuretic response is unknown.

Bumetanide is a newer member of the high-ceiling, or loop, diuretics, which include furosemide and ethacrynic acid. The anatomic site in the nephron for its diuretic effects is the cortical and medullary portions of the ascending limb of the loop of Henle. Bumetanide blocks sodium chloride reabsorption and promotes the urinary excretion of sodium, chloride, potassium, and water from the body.

Metolazone, a thiazide-related compound, appears to inhibit sodium chloride reabsorption in the distal tubule. The urinary excretion pattern is similar to that of the thiazide diuretics, promoting a net loss of sodium, chloride, potassium, and water.

390–391. The answers are: 390-D, 391-B. *(DiPalma, 3/e. pp 414, 417–418. Gilman, 8/e. pp 716–718, 723.)* The oral or parenteral administration of acetazolamide (Diamox), a carbonic anhydrase inhibitor, reduces intraocular pressure in patients who have glaucoma by reducing the rate of aqueous humor formation. Carbonic anhydrase is believed to play a part in aqueous humor secretion. Acetazolamide is a sulfonamide derivative that has been studied most often for its uses as a diuretic and a carbonic anhydrase inhibitor. The ability of acetazolamide to inhibit the activity of carbonic anhydrase appears to be related to its free $—SO_2NH_2$ group, which is a constituent of all carbonic anhydrase inhibitors.

The loop, or high-ceiling, diuretics, such as ethacrynic acid (Edecrin) or furosemide (Lasix), are readily absorbed from the gastrointestinal tract and demonstrate a very rapid onset of action. In general their actions are independent of changes in acid-base balance, but their duration of action is brief.

392–394. The answers are: 392-F, 393-H, 394-E. *(DiPalma, 3/e. pp 415, 417–419. Gilman, 8/e. pp 715, 725–726.)* Acetazolamide is a carbonic anhydrase inhibitor with its primary site of action at the proximal tubule of the nephron. Acetazolamide promotes a urinary excretion of sodium, potassium, and bicarbonate. There is a decrease in loss of chloride ions. The increased excretion of bicarbonate makes the urine alkaline and may produce metabolic acidosis as a consequence of the loss of bicarbonate from the blood. None of the other diuretic drugs promote a reduction in the excretion of the chloride ion.

The only diuretic agent that has a steroid structure is spironolactone. This potassium-sparing diuretic is a competitive inhibitor of aldosterone, which mediates the reabsorption of sodium ions in the collecting duct.

Mannitol is classified as an osmotic diuretic. It is used to maintain urine flow in such cases as trauma and drug intoxication as well as after surgery. In addition, mannitol is used to reduce pressure and volume of cerebrospinal fluid and pre- and postoperatively for short-term reduction of intraocular pressure. Although acetazolamide is used in the treatment of glaucoma, it is not employed to decrease cerebrospinal fluid pressure.

Gastrointestinal System and Nutrition

- Antacids
  - Sodium bicarbonate
  - Aluminum hydroxide
  - Magnesium hydroxide
  - Calcium carbonate
- H_2 Receptor Antagonists
  - Cimetidine
  - Ranitidine
  - Famotidine
  - Nizatidine
- Proton-Pump Inhibitors
  - Omeprazole (Losec)
- Mucosal Protective Agents
  - Sucralfate
  - Colloidal bismuth compounds—Pepto-Bismol
  - Prostaglandins—misoprostal (Cytotec)
- Promotion of GI Motility
  - Metoclopramide (Reglan)
  - Bethanechol
- Pancreatic Replacement Enzymes
  - Pancrelipase (Pancrease, Cotazyme)
- Laxatives
  - Castor oil
  - Cascara, senna, aloes, phenolphthalein, bisacodyl
  - Stool softeners
    - Mineral oil, glycerine suppositories, dioctyl sodium sulfosuccinate (docusate)
  - Bulk laxatives
    - Hydrophilic colloids
    - Saline cathartics
- Antidiarrheal Drugs
  - Diphenoxylate, loperamide
- Dissolution of Gallstones
  - Chenodeoxycholic acid
  - Ursodiol (ursodeoxycholic acid)
- Chronic Inflammatory Bowel Disease
  - Sulfasalazine
- Portal System Encephalopathy
  - Lactulose
  - Branched chain amino acids
- Vitamins
  - Water soluble
    - Thiamine (B_1)
    - Riboflavin (B_2)
    - Nicotinic acid (niacin)
    - Pyridoxine (B_6)
    - Vitamin C (ascorbic acid)
    - Vitamin B_{12}
    - Folic acid
  - Fat Soluble
    - Vitamin A
    - Vitamin D
    - Vitamin E
    - Vitamin K
- Concept of recommended daily allowances

DIRECTIONS: Each question below contains five suggested responses. Select the **one best** response to each question.

395. Cimetidine slows the metabolism of many drugs because it inhibits the activity of

(A) monoamine oxidase
(B) cytochrome P-450
(C) tyrosine kinase
(D) H^+,K^+-ATPase
(E) phase II glucoronidation reactions

396. The absorption of phosphate is reduced when large and prolonged doses of which of the following antacids are given?

(A) Sodium bicarbonate
(B) Magnesium hydroxide
(C) Magnesium trisilicate
(D) Calcium carbonate
(E) Sucralfate

397. Omeprazole (Losec), a new agent for the promotion of healing of peptic ulcers, has a mechanism of action based on

(A) prostaglandins
(B) gastric secretion
(C) pepsin secretion
(D) H^+,K^+-ATPase
(E) anticholinergic action

398. Which of the following is a stool softener that does NOT decrease absorption of fat-soluble vitamins?

(A) Mineral oil
(B) Castor oil
(C) Docusate sodium (Colace)
(D) Phenolphthalein
(E) Cascara sagrada

399. An effective antidiarrheal agent that inhibits peristaltic movement is

(A) clonidine
(B) bismuth subsalicylate
(C) oral electrolyte solution
(D) atropine
(E) diphenoxylate

400. The approved indication for misoprostal (Cytotec) is

(A) reflux esophagitis
(B) healing of gastric ulcer
(C) healing of duodenal ulcer
(D) prevention of gastric ulceration in patients using large doses of aspirin-like drugs
(E) pathologic hypersecretory conditions such as Zollinger-Ellison syndrome

401. True statements concerning sucralfate include all the following EXCEPT

(A) it contains polyaluminum hydroxide
(B) it maintains gel-like qualities even at acid pH
(C) it binds to ulcer craters more than to normal mucosa
(D) it has moderate acid-neutralizing properties
(E) it reacts very little with mucin

402. Metoclopramide (Reglan) has antiemetic properties because it

(A) accelerates gastric emptying time
(B) lowers esophageal sphincter pressure
(C) is a CNS dopamine receptor antagonist
(D) has cholinomimetic properties
(E) has sedative properties

403. The steatorrhea of pancreatic insufficiency can best be treated by

(A) cimetidine
(B) misoprostal
(C) bile salts
(D) pancrelipase
(E) secretin

404. Cholesterol gallstones may be dissolved by oral treatment with

(A) lovastatin
(B) dehydrocholic acid
(C) methyl tertiary butyl ether
(D) chenodeoxycholic acid
(E) monoctanoin

405. A drug of choice in the therapy of inflammatory bowel disease is

(A) sulfadiazine
(B) sulfasalazine
(C) sulfapyridine
(D) sulfamethoxazole
(E) salicylate sodium

406. An important drug in the therapy of portal systemic encephalopathy is

(A) lactulose
(B) lactate
(C) loperamide
(D) lorazepam
(E) loxapine

407. Which of the following commonly used drugs causes overstimulation of the intestinal tract?

(A) Aluminum hydroxide
(B) Trihexyphenidyl
(C) Ferrous sulfate
(D) Chlorpromazine
(E) Bethanechol

408. Bismuth subsalicylate (Pepto-Bismol), a widely used over-the-counter remedy for gastric distress and diarrhea, is apt to produce on long-term administration which of the following complications?

(A) Parkinsonism
(B) Intestinal colic
(C) Dark line at gum margin
(D) Encephalopathy
(E) Psychosis

409. Misoprostol (Cytotec) is contraindicated in

(A) renal impairment
(B) infertility
(C) pregnancy
(D) lactating females
(E) children

410. The primary pharmacologic action of omeprazole (Losec) is reduction of

(A) volume of gastric juice
(B) gastric motility
(C) secretion of pepsin
(D) secretion of gastric acid
(E) secretion of intrinsic factor

411. Which of the following vitamins in large doses is teratogenic?

(A) Vitamin A
(B) Vitamin B_{12}
(C) Vitamin C
(D) Vitamin D
(E) Vitamin E

412. Fat-soluble vitamins have generally a greater potential toxicity compared with water-soluble vitamins because they are

(A) more essential to vital metabolic processes
(B) metabolically faster
(C) avidly stored by the body
(D) administered in larger doses
(E) involved in more essential metabolic pathways

413. In the United States the "Recommended Daily Allowances (RDAs)" are periodically developed by the

(A) National Academy of Sciences
(B) Food and Drug Administration
(C) Department of Agriculture
(D) Department of Commerce
(E) Surgeon General

414. Which vitamin needs to be given in supplemental doses in order to prevent deficiency when a patient is given prolonged administration of isoniazid?

(A) Vitamin A
(B) Vitamin K
(C) Vitamin C
(D) Thiamine
(E) Pyridoxine

DIRECTIONS: Each group of questions below consists of lettered headings followed by a set of numbered items. For each numbered item select the **one** lettered heading with which it is **most** closely associated. Each lettered heading may be used **once, more than once, or not at all.**

Questions 415–419

Match each vitamin with the appropriate description.

(A) Excess amounts should be avoided when the patient is on levodopa
(B) Overdosage may lead to a psychotic state
(C) Improvement of vision especially in daylight might be attributable to this vitamin
(D) This vitamin is usually not included in the popular "one-a-day" vitamin preparations
(E) Retinoic acid is the natural form
(F) Acute intoxication with this vitamin causes hypertension, nausea and vomiting, and signs of increased CSF pressure
(G) This vitamin has hormonal functions
(H) This fat-soluble vitamin has mainly antioxidant properties
(I) In its water-soluble form, this fat-soluble vitamin is capable of producing kernicterus

415. Phytonadione

416. Calcitriol

417. Pyridoxine

418. Menadione

419. Alpha-tocopherol

Questions 420–424

For each vitamin, match the appropriate use or deficiency.

(A) Large doses are used to treat hyperlipoproteinemia
(B) Large doses are used to acidify urine
(C) This vitamin is used in the therapy of Wernicke's syndrome
(D) Large doses are used to cure psychosis
(E) Deficiency can cause angular stomatitis
(F) Deficiency can cause the common cold
(G) Deficiency can cause convulsions in children

420. Riboflavin

421. Nicotinic acid

422. Vitamin C

423. Pyridoxine

424. Thiamine

Gastrointestinal System and Nutrition

Answers

395. The answer is B. *(DiPalma, 3/e. p 179. Gilman, 8/e. p 901.)* Cimetidine reversibly inhibits cytochrome P-450. This is important in phase I biotransformation reactions and inhibits the metabolism of such drugs as warfarin, phenytoin, propranolol, metoprolol, quinidine, and theophylline. None of the other enzymes are significantly affected.

396. The answer is D. *(Gilman, 8/e. p 9. Katzung, 4/e. pp 793–794.)* Although aluminum hydroxide is generally considered to be the antacid that inhibits phosphate absorption, calcium carbonate is equally capable of this effect. This adverse effect may be hazardous in the presence of renal impairment.

397. The answer is D. *(AMA Drug Evaluations Annual 1991, 7/e. pp 783–784. Gilman, 8/e. pp 902–904.)* Omeprozole inhibits H^+,K^+-ATPase, which effectively stops the proton pump and thus prevents the formation of gastric acid. It is the most effective agent in severe cases of ulceration and esophageal reflux.

398. The answer is C. *(Gilman, 8/e. p 922. Katzung, 4/e. p 798.)* Dioctyl sodium sulfosuccinate (docusate) is a detergent that, when given orally, softens the stool and prevents straining. Mineral oil also softens the stool, but it tends to inhibit absorption of fat-soluble vitamins and other nutrients. Castor oil, phenolphthalein, and cascara are strong laxatives and cause watery stools.

399. The answer is E. *(Gilman, 8/e. pp 924–925. Katzung, 4/e. p 798.)* Diphenoxylate is a piperidine opioid related to meperidine. It inhibits peristalsis and hence increases the passage time of the intestinal bolus. It is combined with atropine to discourage use as a street drug. Atropine has little effect on peristalsis. Clonidine, bismuth subsalicylate, and rehydration therapy are all useful in some types of diarrhea, but none of them inhibit peristalsis.

400. The answer is D. *(AMA Drug Evaluations Annual 1991, 7/e. p 783. Gilman, 8/e. p 911.)* Misoprostal is a prostaglandin E analogue that has antisecretory and mucosal protection properties in the stomach. Experimentally it protects against mucosal damage from NSAIDs, alcohol, and other toxic agents. It will also tend to heal existing ulcers but is inferior to other agents in this regard.

401. The answer is D. *(Gilman, 8/e. p 910. Katzung, 4/e. p 796.)* Sucralfate is a sulfated disaccharide that contains polyaluminum hydroxide. It has primarily protective properties and attaches firmly to ulcer craters. It has no significant acid-neutralizing properties.

402. The answer is C. *(Gilman, 8/e. pp 926–928. Katzung, 4/e. pp 796–797.)* Metoclopramide antagonizes the emetic effect of apomorphine, which is mediated by a dopamine receptor in the CNS. It also raises the lower esophageal sphincter pressure and relaxes the pyloric sphincter, which hastens gastric emptying time. This makes it useful in the therapy of reflux esophagitis.

403. The answer is D. *(Gilman, 8/e. pp 929–930. Katzung, 4/e. p 797.)* Pancrelipase (Pancrease, Cotazym) is an alcoholic extract of hog pancreas that contains lipase, trypsin, and amylase. It is effective in reducing the steatorrhea of pancreatic insufficiency. None of the other drugs mentioned have significant action in the digestion of fats.

404. The answer is D. *(Gilman, 8/e. pp 930–931. Katzung, 4/e. pp 798–799.)* Chenodeoxycholic acid (chenodiol) and ursodiol have proved to be effective in some patients with cholesterol gallstones. Lovastatin lowers blood cholesterol levels but has no effect on gallstones. Methyl tertiary butyl ether and a new agent, monoctanoin, are infused directly into the common duct and will dissolve gallstones.

405. The answer is B. *(Gilman, 8/e. p 1051. Katzung, 4/e. p 799.)* Sulfasalazine consists of sulfapyridine with 5-aminosalicylic acid linked by an azo bond. This bond is broken by bacteria that release the salicylic acid, which is believed to be the active agent. Sulfa drugs or salicylic acid used alone is not as effective. The mechanism of action is unknown but is believed to be protective action on the mucosa.

406. The answer is A. *(Gilman, 8/e. pp 919–920. Katzung, 4/e. p 799.)* Lactulose is a synthetic disaccharide (galactose-fructose) that is not absorbed. In moderate doses it acts as a laxative. In higher doses it is capable of binding ammonia and other toxins that form in the intestine in severe liver deficiency and that are believed to cause the encephalopathy. Loperamide is an antidiarrheal opioid; lorazepam is a CNS depressant; loxapine is a tricyclic antipsychotic.

407. The answer is E. *(DiPalma, 3/e. p 131. Gilman, 8/e. p 916.)* Bethanechol, a cholinomimetic drug, has selectivity for the urogenital tract, but frequent adverse reactions include abdominal cramping and even involuntary defecation. Trihexyphenidyl, an antiparkinsonism drug, and chlorpromazine, an antipsychotic, have anticholinergic action that depresses intestinal function. Ferrous sulfate and aluminum hydroxide are constipative.

408. The answer is D. *(DiPalma, 3/e. p 698. Gilman, 8/e. p 910.)* Colloidal bismuth salts are poorly absorbed, but on long-term use the bismuth blood level does rise. The most common complication is encephalopathy. A so-called lead gum line does not occur, although darkening of the mouth may eventually occur. Manganese may cause parkinsonism; intestinal colic is caused by lead; and psychosis is caused by mercury.

409. The answer is C. *(AMA Drug Evaluations Annual 1991, 7/e. p 783. Gilman, 8/e. p 911.)* The only absolute contraindication to the use of misoprostol is pregnancy or in women of childbearing age. Prostaglandins are abortifacients. Although there is evidence in animals that prostaglandins impair fertility, it is unlikely that misoprostol would decrease human fertility. Misoprostol is rapidly metabolized and does not concentrate in the milk. Use in renal impairment requires caution. Although misoprostol is not approved for use in children, it is used and there are no apparent ill effects.

410. The answer is D. *(AMA Drug Evaluations Annual 1991, 7/e. pp 783–784. Gilman, 8/e. p 903.)* The main action of omeprazole is inhibition of secretion of gastric acid. Because it is a specific inhibitor of the proton pump (H^+,K^+-ATPase), other actions are secondary to the marked decline of acid secretion. As a result of the reduction of gastric acidity, there is increased secretion of gastrin leading to hypergastrinemia.

411. The answer is A. *(AMA Drug Evaluations Annual 1991, 7/e. pp 1871–1872. Gilman, 8/e. p 1559.)* Pregnant women should not take more than a 25 percent increase in the normal dietary intake of vitamin A for it is definitely teratogenic, especially in the first trimester of pregnancy. Great caution is to be taken in premenopausal females in the therapy of acne and skin wrinkling in which tretinoin or isotretinoin is the therapeutic agent. None of the other vitamins is particularly teratogenic except perhaps vitamin D.

412. The answer is C. *(AMA Drug Evaluations Annual 1991, 7/e. pp 1871–1875. Gilman, 8/e. p 1524.)* Fat-soluble vitamins, especially vitamins A and D, can be stored in massive amounts and hence have a potential for serious toxicities. Water-soluble vitamins are easily excreted by the kidney and toxic accumulation rarely occurs.

413. The answer is A. *(AMA Drug Evaluations Annual 1991, 7/e. p 1868. Gilman, 8/e. p 1524.)* The National Academy of Sciences has a Food and Nutrition Board, which has the function of selecting the levels of vitamins, minerals, and other substances necessary to achieve maximum nutritional health. The levels are reviewed periodically and determined by study of the nutritional needs of healthy persons. The Food and Drug Administration is responsible for labeling of nutritional products but does not determine the RDAs.

414. The answer is E. *(DiPalma, 3/e. p 627. Katzung, 4/e. p 579.)* The toxicity of isoniazid (INH) is mainly on the peripheral and central nervous systems. This is attributable to competition of INH with pyridoxal phosphate for apotryptophanase. This results in a relative deficiency of pyridoxine, which causes peripheral neuritis, insomnia, and muscle twitching among other effects.

415–419. The answers are: 415-D, 416-G, 417-A, 418-I, 419-H. *(DiPalma, 3/e. pp 414–415, 490–495. Gilman, 8/e. pp 1523–1570.)* Phytonadione, the fat-soluble form of vitamin K, is usually not included in so-called one-a-day vitamin preparations because it is so ubiquitous in the usual diet. Only in liver disease does a deficiency of the vitamin occur.

Calcitriol (1,25-D_3) is the most active form of vitamin D. It is formed by the kidney. When the calcium blood level rises, the kidney produces 24,25-D_3, a much less active form. Vitamin D can be manufactured in the body by the action of sunlight on the skin. Its main action is to increase calcium absorption in the gut. Thus, vitamin D subserves important hormonal functions in calcium homeostasis.

Levodopa is converted to dopamine in the peripheral tissues by dopa decarboxylase, which has as a cofactor pyridoxine. Excess of this vitamin will increase this reaction, which is an undesirable effect because dopamine does not cross the blood-brain barrier where the therapeutic effect is desired.

Menadione, the water-soluble form of vitamin K, should not be given to infants because of the high incidence of hemolysis and jaundice.

Alpha-tocopherol, or vitamin E, is relatively nontoxic and has antioxidant properties, e.g., preserving intracellular components such as ubiquinone.

420–424. The answers are: 420-E, 421-A, 422-B, 423-G, 424-C. *(AMA Drug Evaluations Annual 1991, 7/e. pp 1875–1880. Gilman, 8/e. pp 1523–1570.)* Angular stomatitis, dermatitis, and corneal vascularization are considered classic signs of human riboflavin deficiency, although multiple B vitamins may be involved.

Nicotinic acid (niacin) in doses of 1 to 3 g a day, over 100 times the RDA, causes a significant lowering of blood cholesterol. This is not an attribute of nicotinamide. Nicotinic acid and nicotinamide are both effective in curing pellagra. Large doses of nicotinic acid have been used in attempts to cure various psychoses, but this therapy is now discredited.

Vitamin C, which is sometimes recommended in large doses for the common cold and as a cure for cancer, is actually more useful as a method of acidifying urine and increasing the excretion of such abused drugs as phencyclidine.

Pyridoxine deficiency is most common in children on infant formulas that do not contain this vitamin. Deficiency of this vitamin causes convulsions.

The classic therapy of the bizarre CNS signs and symptoms of withdrawal in severe alcoholics is intravenous administration of thiamine plus glucose infusion. Alcoholics generally have other deficiencies of vitamins, especially riboflavin and niacin.

Endocrine System

Anabolic Steroids
- Dromostanolone propionate
- Methandrostenolone
- Nandrolone decanoate
- Nandrolone phenpropionate
- Oxandrolone
- Oxymetholone
- Stanozolol

Corticosteroids
- Beclomethasone
- Cortisone
- Dexamethasone
- Fludrocortisone
- Hydrocortisone
- Prednisone*
- Methylprednisolone
- Metyrapone
- Spironolactone
- Triamcinolone

Corticotropins
- Corticotropin (ACTH)*
- Cosyntropin

Female Sex Hormones and Oral Contraceptives
- Chlorotrianisene*
- Conjugated estrogens
- Danazol*
- Dienestrol
- Diethylstilbestrol
- Estradiol
- Estrone
- Ethinyl estradiol
- Ethynodiol
- Hydroxyprogesterone
- Leuprolide*
- Levonorgestrel
- Luteinizing hormone–releasing hormone
- Medroxyprogesterone
- Megestrol
- Mestranol
- Norethindrone
- Norethynodrel
- Norgestrel
- Quinestrol
- Tamoxifen*

Fertility Agents
- Bromocriptine*
- Clomiphene*
- Human chorionic gonadotropin (hCG)
- Human menopausal gonadotropin (hMG)

Hyperglycemic Agents
- Diazoxide
- Glucagon*

Insulins
- Extended insulin zinc suspension
- Insulin injection
- Insulin zinc suspension
- Isophane (NPH)
- Prompt insulin zinc suspension
- Protamine zinc insulin suspension

Male Sex Hormones
- Fluoxymesterone
- Methyltestosterone*
- Testosterone*
- Testosterone cypionate
- Testosterone enanthate
- Testosterone propionate

Oral Hypoglycemic Agents
- Acetohexamide
- Chlorpropamide
- Glipizide
- Glyburide
- Tolazamide
- Tolbutamide*

Parathyroid Drugs
- Calcitonin*
- Calcitriol
- Calcifediol
- Dihydrotachysterol
- Ergocalciferol
- Etidronate*
- Parathyroid hormone (PTH)
- Phosphates
- Plicamycin (mithramycin)
- Vitamin D*

Thyroid Drugs
- Dessicated thyroid*
- Iodide (Lugol's solution)
- Levothyroxine
- Liothyronine
- Liotrix
- Methimazole
- Propylthiouracil*
- Protirelin
- Radioactive iodine (^{131}I)

DIRECTIONS: Each question below contains five suggested responses. Select the **one best** response to each question.

425. Triamcinolone (Aristocort) can produce which one of the following effects?

(A) Enhanced glycogenolysis
(B) Increased amino acid content of muscle
(C) Redistribution of body fat
(D) Lowered serum glucose levels
(E) Inhibition of glucagon secretion

426. Drugs that bind to receptors in the plasma membrane and enhance levels of cyclic 3′,5′-adenosine monophosphate (cAMP) include all the following EXCEPT

(A) adrenocorticotropic hormone (ACTH)
(B) calcitonin
(C) isoproterenol
(D) hydrocortisone
(E) glucagon

427. A patient with diarrhea, nausea, dermatitis, and psychic disturbances is probably deficient in which of the following vitamins?

(A) Pyridoxine
(B) Thiamine
(C) Pantothenic acid
(D) Niacin (nicotinic acid)
(E) Ascorbic acid

428. True statements about testosterone include all the following EXCEPT

(A) it is biotransformed primarily in the liver
(B) it enhances the excretion of sodium and water
(C) it has a stimulatory effect on hematopoietic cells
(D) it attaches to a receptor on the X chromosome
(E) it is converted to an active metabolite, dihydrotestosterone (DHT)

429. True statements concerning triiodothyronine (T_3) or thyroxine (T_4) include all the following EXCEPT

(A) T_3 readily penetrates cellular membrane
(B) T_3 attaches to cytoplasmic binders
(C) halogenase converts T_4 to T_3
(D) T_3 binds to receptors in the nucleus
(E) T_4 is actively transported into the cell

430. A substance that enhances the probability of ovulation by blocking the inhibitory effect of estrogens and thus stimulating the release of gonadotropin from the pituitary is

(A) oxymetholone
(B) clomiphene (Clomid)
(C) diethylstilbestrol
(D) ethinyl estradiol
(E) progesterone

431. A naturally occurring substance useful in treating Paget's disease of bone is

(A) etidronate
(B) cortisol
(C) calcitonin
(D) parathyroid hormone
(E) thyroxine

432. The requirement for thiamine is greatest under which of the following conditions?

(A) Stressful procedures
(B) Consumption of megadoses of vitamin C
(C) High-fat diet
(D) High-protein diet
(E) High-carbohydrate diet

433. The preferred thyroid preparation for maintenance replacement therapy is which of the following drugs?

(A) Desiccated thyroid
(B) Liothyronine (Cytomel)
(C) Protirelin (Thypinone)
(D) Levothyroxine (Levothroid)
(E) Liotrix (Euthroid)

434. A patient becomes markedly tetanic following a recent thyroidectomy. This symptom can be rapidly reversed by the administration of

(A) vitamin D
(B) calcitonin
(C) parathyroid hormone
(D) plicamycin (mithramycin)
(E) calcium gluconate

435. Inhibition of the peripheral conversion of T_4 to T_3 by the liver and kidney is caused by all the following drugs EXCEPT

(A) propranolol (Inderal)
(B) amiodarone (Cordarone)
(C) hydrocortisone
(D) methimazole (Tapazole)
(E) propylthiouracil (PTU)

436. The steroid having the LEAST mineralocorticoid potency is which of the following?

(A) Cortisone
(B) Fludrocortisone
(C) Spironolactone
(D) 11-Desoxycorticosterone
(E) Hydrocortisone

437. All the following are steroid compounds EXCEPT

(A) mestranol
(B) clomiphene (Clomid)
(C) ethynodiol diacetate (Demulen)
(D) norethindrone (Norlutin)
(E) beclomethasone

438. Metyrapone is useful in testing the endocrine functioning of the

(A) α cells of pancreatic islets
(B) β cells of pancreatic islets
(C) neurohypophysis
(D) pituitary-adrenal axis
(E) Leydig cells of testes

439. True statements about dexamethasone (Decadron) include all the following EXCEPT

(A) it can stimulate lung maturation in the fetus
(B) it is used for the diagnosis of Cushing's syndrome
(C) it has minimal mineralocorticoid activity
(D) it is a short-acting glucocorticoid
(E) it is potentially ulcerogenic

440. Abuse of anabolic steroids by athletes can result in all the following EXCEPT

(A) retention of fluid
(B) feminization in males
(C) decreased spermatogenesis
(D) depression
(E) anorexia

441. Drugs that increase the need for insulin include all the following EXCEPT

(A) epinephrine
(B) hydrocortisone
(C) chlorthalidone (Hygroton)
(D) dexamethasone (Decadron)
(E) ethanol (acute ingestion)

442. Which of the following is the insulin preparation with the longest duration of action?

(A) Insulin injection (regular insulin)
(B) Prompt insulin zinc suspension (Semilente)
(C) Isophane insulin suspension (NPH insulin)
(D) Insulin zinc suspension (Lente)
(E) Protamine zinc insulin suspension (PZI)

443. Bromocriptine (Parlodel) is used to treat some cases of amenorrhea because it

(A) stimulates release of gonadotropin-releasing hormone
(B) stimulates the ovary directly
(C) is an estrogen antagonist that enhances gonadotropin release
(D) inhibits prolactin release
(E) increases the synthesis of follicle-stimulating hormone

444. The general structure for thyroid hormones is shown below. In order for this structure to acquire significant hormone activity, all the following modifications must take place EXCEPT that

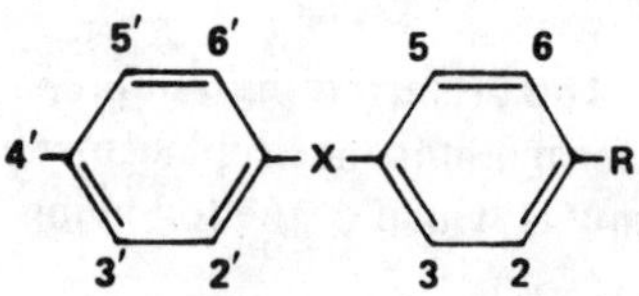

(A) the connection between the two aromatic rings should be by ether, thioether, or methylene linkage
(B) the R side chain on carbon 1 should be aliphatic and contain a carboxyl group
(C) halogenation or methylation is necessary at positions 3 and 5
(D) a hydroxyl group should be on position 3′
(E) position 4′ should have a hydroxyl group or a group capable of being metabolically converted to hydroxyl

445. Tamoxifen is used to treat some breast cancers because of its ability to

(A) utilize its androgenic properties in retarding tumor growth
(B) prevent estrogen synthesis by the ovary
(C) enhance glucocorticoid treatment
(D) act as an estrogen antagonist
(E) act as a potent progestin

446. Drugs that enter the cytoplasm of a cell and then bind to a specific receptor include all the following EXCEPT

(A) trihexyphenidyl (Artane)
(B) triamcinolone (Aristocort)
(C) mestranol
(D) fludrocortisone (Florinef)
(E) calcitriol (Rocaltrol)

447. Which one of the following statements is true of oxytocin?

(A) It is used for postpartum bleeding
(B) It is approved for use in elective induction of labor
(C) Overdosage can cause a sustained tetanic contraction
(D) It causes a large increase in blood pressure
(E) It inhibits milk ejection

448. The most dangerous adverse reaction to the administration of methimazole (Tapazole) is

(A) hypothyroidism
(B) arthralgia
(C) jaundice
(D) agranulocytosis
(E) renal toxicity

449. True statements about calcitriol (Rocaltrol) include all the following EXCEPT

(A) it is formed in the kidney from calcifediol by hydroxylation
(B) it may cause arrhythmias in digitalized patients
(C) it has a rapid onset of action
(D) it is 25-OH_3-vitamin D_3
(E) it enhances intestinal absorption of calcium

450. Symptoms of vitamin A deficiency include all the following EXCEPT

(A) decreased intracranial pressure
(B) keratomalacia
(C) night blindness
(D) cancellous bone formation
(E) follicular hyperkeratosis

451. Adverse reactions to norethindrone include all the following EXCEPT

(A) acne
(B) weight gain
(C) hirsutism
(D) cholestatic jaundice
(E) venous thromboembolic disease

452. The treatment of myxedema coma can include which of the following agents?

(A) Thyroglobulin
(B) Levothyroxine
(C) Lithium
(D) Propylthiouracil
(E) Protirelin (Relefact TRH)

453. The "minipill" containing only a progestin, rather than a combination estrogen-progestin oral contraceptive, was developed because progestin alone

(A) results in less depression and cholestatic jaundice
(B) is a more effective contraceptive agent than the two combined
(C) results in a more regular menstrual cycle
(D) is thought to be less likely to induce endometriosis
(E) is thought to be less likely to induce cardiovascular disorders

454. Parathyroid hormone has which one of the following effects?

(A) Increased mobilization of calcium from bone
(B) Decreased active absorption of calcium from the small intestine
(C) Decreased renal tubular reabsorption of calcium
(D) Decreased resorption of phosphate from bone
(E) Decreased excretion of phosphate

455. Adverse reactions to administration of chlorpropamide (Diabinese) include all the following EXCEPT

(A) water retention
(B) increased tolerance to ethanol
(C) hypoglycemia
(D) hyponatremia
(E) exacerbation of peptic ulcers

456. True statements about danazol (Danocrine) include all the following EXCEPT

(A) it is a testosterone derivative
(B) it can cause edema
(C) it can cause gynecomastia
(D) it can decrease HDL cholesterol
(E) it is indicated in endometriosis

457. Hypervitaminosis D produces all the following effects EXCEPT

(A) nephrocalcinosis
(B) polyuria
(C) osteoporosis
(D) polydipsia
(E) mild alkalosis

458. Adverse reactions associated with methylprednisolone include all the following EXCEPT

(A) osteoporosis
(B) peptic ulceration
(C) increased susceptibility to infection
(D) hypoglycemia
(E) edema

459. True statements about glyburide include all the following EXCEPT

(A) it is mildly diuretic
(B) it promotes the release of insulin
(C) it is a second-generation oral hypoglycemic agent
(D) its duration of action is 12 to 24 h and the drug may be given once a day
(E) it may decrease tolerance to ethanol

460. All the following drugs can cause hyperglycemia and hypokalemia EXCEPT

(A) hydrocortisone
(B) chlorpropamide
(C) hydrochlorothiazide
(D) bumetanide
(E) prednisone

DIRECTIONS: Each group of questions below consists of lettered headings followed by a set of numbered items. For each numbered item select the **one** lettered heading with which it is **most** closely associated. Each lettered heading may be used **once, more than once, or not at all.**

Questions 461–464

Match each clinical use or entity below with the most appropriate drug.

(A) Ethinyl estradiol
(B) Spironolactone (Aldactone)
(C) Aminoglutethimide (Cytadren)
(D) Leuprolide
(E) Fludrocortisone (Florinef)

461. "Morning-after" contraception

462. Primary hyperaldosteronism

463. Mineralocorticoid replacement therapy in primary adrenal insufficiency

464. Advanced prostate cancer

Questions 465–468

For each inhibitory effect on the synthesis of thyroid hormone listed below, select the agent that causes it.

(A) Sodium thiocyanate
(B) Methimazole (Tapazole)
(C) Triiodothyronine
(D) Radioactive iodine
(E) Iodide

465. Inhibits, by acting as a competitor, the accumulation of iodide in thyroid follicular cells

466. Inhibits the peroxidase-catalyzed oxidation of iodide and thus interferes with the incorporation of iodide into an organic structure

467. Inhibits the peroxidase-catalyzed coupling of iodotyrosines to form iodothyronines

468. Inhibits the secretion of thyroid hormone

Questions 469–471

Select the drug most likely to produce each effect.

(A) Acetohexamide
(B) Chlorpropamide
(C) Calcitriol
(D) Diazoxide
(E) Etidronate
(F) Glyburide
(G) Liotrix
(H) Methimazole
(I) Primidone
(J) Propylthiouracil

469. Inhibits the conversion of tetraiodothyronine (T_4) to triiodothyronine (T_3)

470. Inhibits the secretion of insulin

471. Inhibits bone resorption

Questions 472–474

Match each statement with the correct drug.

(A) Aldosterone
(B) Clomiphene
(C) Diazoxide
(D) Fludrocortisone
(E) Isophane insulin
(F) Methimazole
(G) Ethinyl estradiol
(H) Norethindrone
(I) Norethynodrel
(J) Propylthiouracil
(K) Salicylates
(L) Spironolactone
(M) Tamoxifen
(N) Triamcinolone

472. This drug promotes the synthesis of factors II, VII, IX, and X and may interfere with the effect of warfarin or may result in thromboembolic phenomena

473. The therapeutic effect of this drug is reduced by glucocorticoids, dextrothyroxine, epinephrine, hydrochlorothiazide, and levothyroxine

474. This drug reduces the growth of facial hair in idiopathic hirsutism or hirsutism secondary to androgen excess

Endocrine System

Answers

425. The answer is C. *(DiPalma, 3/e. pp 540–541. Katzung, 4/e. pp 482–486.)* The administration of a glucocorticoid compound such as triamcinolone or hydrocortisone causes an elevation in serum glucose levels by decreasing peripheral utilization of glucose, increasing gluconeogenesis, and possibly stimulating the secretion of glucagon. There is suppression of protein synthesis in skeletal muscle and a decreased content of amino acids. Amino acids are converted to glucose by hepatic gluconeogenesis. Large doses of corticosteroid appear to increase lipogenesis and lipolysis in certain areas of the body with a redistribution of fat. There is a reduction of fat content of the legs and arms and an enhancement of supraclavicular areas.

426. The answer is D. *(DiPalma, 3/e. pp 21–25, 27–29, 535, 537–540.)* Cyclic AMP is an intracellular second messenger that is involved in the mechanism of action associated with adrenocorticotropic hormone, calcitonin, isoproterenol, and glucagon. These agents complex with a plasma membrane receptor that brings about the binding of guanosine triphosphate (GTP) to the coupling protein and the activation of adenylate cyclase. Adenylate cyclase catalyzes the formation of cAMP from ATP. In the cytoplasm cAMP activates cAMP-dependent protein kinase, which participates in the phosphorylation of specific substrate proteins (e.g., enzymes). The phosphorylated protein eventually induces the particular response on the target cell that is associated with the administered drug. The cellular mechanism of action of hydrocortisone, a glucocorticoid, is also related to proteins but not by the enhancement of cAMP production. Hydrocortisone is transported by simple diffusion across the membrane of the cell into the cytoplasm and binds to a specific receptor. The steroid-receptor complex is activated and enters the nucleus, where it regulates transcription of specific gene sequences into RNA. Eventually mRNA is translated to form specific proteins in the cytoplasm that are involved in the steroid-induced cellular response.

427. The answer is D. *(Gilman, 8/e. pp 1536–1538.)* Niacin, or nicotinic acid, is converted into NAD and NADP, which are necessary for a variety of oxidation-reduction enzyme reactions. Tryptophan may be used instead of nicotinic acid to synthesize the coenzymes. A deficiency of niacin causes pellagra, characterized by diarrhea and gastrointestinal disturbances, dermatitis, and dementia.

428. The answer is B. *(DiPalma, 3/e. pp 528–530, 532. Katzung, 4/e. pp 509–510.)* In many tissues testosterone is transformed into dihydrotestosterone (DHT) by 5α-reductase. This active metabolite is more potent than testosterone and appears to be responsible for the androgenic effects in the body. The affinity of dihydrostestosterone is 10 times that of testosterone for the androgen-receptor gene that is located on the X chromosome. The compound testosterone is eliminated from the body through biotransformation in the liver and excretion of its metabolites, 17-ketosteroids, in the urine. Adverse reactions of testosterone and its various derivatives include virilism in prepubertal males and masculinization in females. Some other untoward effects are liver dysfunction, hypercalcemia, and retention of sodium and water. Therapeutic uses of androgenic compounds are in the area of male hypogonadism, certain types of breast carcinomas, and anemia. Androgens are used in some forms of anemia because they cause the release of erythropoietic-stimulating factor, which increases production of red blood cells.

429. The answer is E. *(DiPalma, 3/e. p 486. Katzung, 4/e. p 468.)* The receptors that bind the physiologic ligand of thyroid hormone appear to be located in the nucleus of the cell as opposed to the cytoplasmic location of steroid receptors. Both T_4 and T_3 enter the cell in the same manner, which is probably by passive diffusion. In the cytoplasm halogenase converts T_4 to T_3. T_3 can attach to cytoplasmic binders or enter the nucleus and bind to receptors. The T_3-receptor complex in association with DNA eventually directs the synthesis of new protein, which changes cellular activity to reflect the presence of thyroid hormone.

430. The answer is B. *(DiPalma, 3/e. pp 516–517. Katzung, 4/e. pp 507–508.)* Clomiphene (Clomid) is an effective fertility drug that can lead to multiple pregnancies. Clomiphene has been termed an antiestrogen because its stimulant effect on the secretion of pituitary gonadotropins is thought to be the consequence of its blocking the inhibitory effect of estrogens on gonadotropin secretion. Side effects of this drug can include alopecia, breast engorgement, and hot flashes. Oxymetholone is an orally effective anabolic steroid.

431. The answer is C. *(DiPalma, 3/e. pp 492–493. Gilman, 8/e. pp 1507–1510. Katzung, 4/e. pp 534–535.)* Calcitonin is useful in the therapy of Paget's disease of bone (osteitis deformans). Calcitonin therapy reduces urinary hydroxyproline excretion and serum alkaline phosphatase activity and provides some symptomatic relief. Presumably these effects result from the ability of calcitonin to inhibit bone resorption. Side effects of long-term therapy with this hormone can include nausea, edema of the hands, and urticaria. The appearance of neutralizing antibodies may explain the development of resistance to treatment. Etidronate is a synthetic drug that is useful in Paget's disease. The compound is orally effective and lacks the antigenicity associated with calcitonin.

432. The answer is E. *(Gilman, 8/e. pp 1530–1534.)* Thiamine pyrophosphate is formed from thiamine and acts as a coenzyme in the decarboxylation of α-ketoglutarate and pyruvate, as well as the hexose monophosphate shunt. Therefore, it is an important part of carbohydrate metabolism. Patients who are being maintained on dextrose need extra amounts of the vitamin. Under normal circumstances, 1 mg per day is recommended.

433. The answer is D. *(AMA Drug Evaluations Annual 1991, 7/e. p 855. DiPalma, 3/e. pp 487–489.)* The drug of choice for maintenance replacement therapy of hypothyroidism is levothyroxine (T_4). Monitoring of plasma blood levels of T_3 and T_4 from the administration of levothyroxine causes less difficulty than the monitoring of plasma hormone levels from liothyronine (T_3), since considerable fluctuation can occur with plasma concentrations of T_3. In addition T_3 has a shorter half-life. Liotrix is a mixture of T_4 and T_3 in a ratio of 4:1 that is designed to resemble the physiologic secretion of the thyroid gland. When liotrix is administered, the T_4 component is converted to T_3 in the body, and T_3, therefore, is actually not needed. It does not appear that liotrix provides any therapeutic advantage over levothyroxine by itself for the usual treatment of hypothyroidism. The treatment of hypothyroidism with desiccated thyroid is obsolete. Protirelin, a synthetic tripeptide, is chemically identical to thyrotropin-releasing hormone (TRH). This compound is used for the diagnosis of mild cases of hypothyroidism or hyperthyroidism.

434. The answer is E. *(Gilman, 8/e. pp 1247, 1507–1517. Katzung, 4/e. pp 535, 538.)* Administration of intravenous calcium gluconate would immediately correct the tetany that might occur in a patient in whom a thyroidectomy was recently performed. Parathyroid hormone would act more slowly but could be given for its future stabilizing effect. Long-term control of a patient after a thyroidectomy can be obtained with vitamin D and dietary therapy. Calcitonin is a hypocalcemic antagonist of parathyroid hormone. Plicamycin (mithramycin) is used to treat Paget's disease and hypercalcemia. The dose employed is about one-tenth the amount used for plicamycin's cytotoxic action.

435. The answer is D. *(AMA Drug Evaluations Annual 1991, 7/e. pp 861–862, 864. DiPalma, 3/e. pp 484–485, 488.)* Triiodothyronine (T_3) and thyroxine (T_4) are released from the thyroid gland and enter the circulation. T_4 is converted to T_3, which is more potent in activity, by the liver and kidney. This conversion reaction is inhibited by propranolol, amiodarone, hydrocortisone, and propylthiouracil. Although methimazole and propylthiouracil inhibit the enzymatic oxidation of iodide ion to active iodine, which is their principal mechanism as antithyroid drugs, only propylthiouracil can block the peripheral conversion of T_4 to T_3. Propranolol and hydrocortisone are used in the treatment of certain cases of hyperthyroidism, and whether the reduction in the conversion of T_4 to T_3 plays a significant role in their mechanism of action is not fully known. The compound amiodarone is an antiarrhythmic drug that is similar in chemical structure to thyroxine. Hypothyroidism and less commonly hyperthyroidism have been reported as adverse reactions to the use of amiodarone.

436. The answer is C. *(DiPalma, 3/e. pp 540, 544–545. Katzung, 4/e. pp 192, 482.)* Steroids that cause the retention of sodium and water by the body are referred to as having mineralocorticoid activity. Fludrocortisone is a potent mineralocorticoid and glucocorticoid compound. Spironolactone interferes with binding of aldosterone, desoxycorticosterone, cortisone, and hydrocortisone to sites in the collecting duct of the nephron. Spironolactone possesses no mineralocorticoid activity and, therefore, will promote a sodium diuresis by competitive inhibition of aldosterone.

437. The answer is B. *(DiPalma, 3/e. pp 513, 516–517, 518. Katzung, 4/e. pp 491, 496, 500.)* All the compounds listed in the question are steroids with the exception of clomiphene (Clomid), an estrogen analogue that lacks the essential feature of a steroid: a hydrogenated cyclopentenophenanthrene-ring system. Clomid is a derivative of the weakly estrogenic compound chlorotrianisene. The compound has high antiestrogenic activity that inhibits estrogenic feedback repression of gonadotropic secretion. Clomid is an effective fertility-inducing drug.

438. The answer is D. *(DiPalma, 3/e. pp 543–544. Katzung, 4/e. p 490.)* Metyrapone (Metopirone), because it decreases serum levels of cortisol by inhibiting the 11β-hydroxylation of steroids in the adrenal, can be used to assess the function of the pituitary-adrenal axis. When metyrapone is administered orally or intravenously to normal persons, the adenohypophysis will secrete an increased amount of adrenocorticotropic hormone (ACTH). This will cause a normal adrenal gland to synthesize increased amounts of 17-hydroxylated steroids that can be measured in the urine. However, patients who have disease of the hypothalamico-pituitary complex are not able to respond to administration of metyrapone by producing increased amounts of ACTH; consequently, no increased levels of 17-hydroxylated steroids would be detected in the urine. Before administering the drug, the ability of the adrenal gland to respond to ACTH must be tested.

439. The answer is D. *(DiPalma, 3/e. pp 543–545. Katzung, 4/e. pp 482–486.)* The compound dexamethasone is classified as a long-acting ($t_{1/2}$ = 36 h) synthetic glucocorticoid. This drug is a 9α-fluoro, 16α-methyl derivative that possesses little or no mineralocorticoid activity. When dexamethasone is compared with hydrocortisone for mineralocorticoid potency at an equivalent dose, dexamethasone is rated as zero, while hydrocortisone is given a value of 1. It is reported that dexamethasone induces ulceration of the gastrointestinal tract. Glucocorticoids appear to stimulate production of acid and pepsin in the stomach. Dexamethasone is used to reduce the occurrence of respiratory distress syndrome in premature infants. This steroid stimulates lung maturation when large doses are given to the mother prior to early delivery. Dexamethasone is also used for diagnostic purposes. The drug is used in the diagnosis of Cushing's syndrome and has been employed in the differential diagnosis of depressive psychiatric states.

440. The answer is E. *(DiPalma, 3/e. p 533. Katzung, 4/e. p 512.)* The use of anabolic steroids by athletes has become quite alarming in recent years. These steroids, which have androgenic and anabolic effects, are used to improve the performance of athletes in various competitive sports. Continued use of anabolic steroids induces mood changes as well as mental disorders from depression to psychosis. The androgenic properties of these drugs cause masculinization in females and may produce feminization in males. This latter effect is due to increased formation of estrogens. In addition, these steroids decrease production of endogenous testosterone by the testes and may cause a reduction in spermatogenesis. The weight gain that occurs with the administration of anabolic steroids may be due to fluid retention and an improved appetite rather than actual tissue growth. These drugs cause liver damage and increase the risk of cardiovascular diseases.

441. The answer is E. *(DiPalma, 3/e. pp 499, 502–503, 540.)* The regulation of levels of blood glucose by insulin and the general effectiveness of insulin are altered with the coadministration of other drugs. Epinephrine enhances glycogenolysis and thereby elevates glucose in the plasma. Glucocorticoids (e.g., hydrocortisone and dexamethasone) stimulate gluconeogenesis, reduce the peripheral utilization of glucose, and decrease the sensitivity of tissues to insulin. Chlorthalidone, a thiazide-related diuretic, may induce hyperglycemia by inhibition of the release of insulin and decrease use of glucose by peripheral tissues. In the presence of ethanol, the effect of insulin is enhanced. When ethanol is acutely ingested in sufficient quantities, the drug causes an alteration in carbohydrate metabolism that results in hypoglycemia. The exact mechanism of the hypoglycemic effect of ethanol has not been fully delineated.

442. The answer is E. *(DiPalma, 3/e. pp 500–502. Gilman, 8/e. pp 1475–1478.)* Insulin injection (also known as *regular,* or *crystalline zinc, insulin*) is effective for about 6 to 8 h; prompt insulin zinc suspension (Semilente) for about 12 to 16 h; isophane insulin suspension (also known as *NPH insulin*) for about 18 to 26 h; insulin zinc suspension (Lente) for about 18 to 26 h; and protamine zinc insulin suspension (PZI) for about 36 h. The last, first prepared in 1936, is a complexed protein that, because of its chemical nature, dissolves slowly at the injection site to allow the insulin to be absorbed slowly and steadily. Extended insulin zinc suspension, also effective for 36 h, is a slowly dissolving insulin and zinc mixture that has no protamine.

443. The answer is D. *(DiPalma, 3/e. p 526. Katzung, 4/e. p 339.)* High prolactin levels in the serum result in amenorrhea, for reasons that are not known. Bromocriptine inhibits prolactin secretion through its dopaminergic action. This compound, a semisynthetic ergot derivative, appears to be a dopamine receptor agonist. It is administered orally to the patient, and in most cases menses occurs after a month of therapy.

444. The answer is D. *(DiPalma, 3/e. p 485. Gilman, 8/e. pp 1361–1365.)* According to extensive research on the relationship between structure and activity of thyronine derivatives, significant thyroid hormone activity would be characteristic of the structure below.

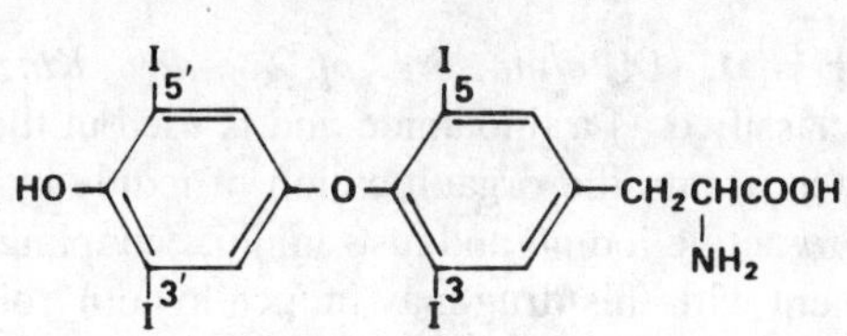

This structure is thyroxine, in which the R side chain is L-alanine, the aromatic rings are connected by an ether linkage, halogenation by iodine occurs on positions 3,5 and 3′,5′, and a hydroxyl group is attached to carbon 4′. Activity can be increased fourfold upon removing iodine from the 5′ position because 3′-monosubstituted compounds have more activity than 3′,5′-disubstituted derivatives of thyronine.

445. The answer is D. *(DiPalma, 3/e. p 516. Gilman, 8/e. pp 1207, 1256–1257.)* Tamoxifen is an estrogen antagonist used in the treatment of breast cancer. Postmenopausal women with metastases to soft tissue and whose tumors contain an estrogen receptor are most likely to respond to this agent. Little benefit is derived from tamoxifen if the tumor does not have estrogen receptors.

446. The answer is A. *(DiPalma, 3/e. pp 27–28, 290, 493, 511–514, 537–540.)* A variety of drugs that resemble steroid hormones in their structure can transverse cellular membranes and bind to specific cytoplasmic receptors. Triamcinolone (a glucocorticoid), fludrocortisone (a mineralocorticoid), mestranol (a sex steroid), and calcitriol (a vitamin D metabolite) all bind reversibly to the cytoplasmic receptor, which then undergoes an irreversible activation step. Next, the steroid-receptor complex enters the nucleus of the cell and regulates transcription of specific genes into RNA. Eventually mRNA is formed and causes the synthesis of specific proteins that mediate the steroid response. The response occurs 30 min to several hours following administration of the drug, since a period of time is required for formation of new proteins in the cell. Trihexyphenidyl is a synthetic anticholinergic drug that binds to muscarinic receptors associated with the cell membrane. This drug is used in the treatment of parkinsonism.

447. The answer is C. *(Gilman, 8/e. pp 935–937, 948. Katzung, 4/e. pp 461–462.)* Oxytocin is used to induce or stimulate medically indicated labor; it should not be used for elective inductions. When used for inductions, it should be administered intravenously so that the rate of infusion can be controlled. If too much oxytocin is administered, a sustained tetanic contraction can result, which may rupture the uterus or cause fetal hypoxia. Oxytocin can cause milk ejection.

448. The answer is D. *(DiPalma, 3/e. pp 488–489. Katzung, 4/e. p 472.)* Methimazole is classified as a thioamide and is used in the treatment of hyperthyroidism. It prevents the organification of iodide by blocking the oxidation of iodide to active iodine and also inhibits coupling of iodotyrosines. Excessive treatment with this drug may induce hypothyroidism. Some other adverse reactions reported for methimazole include skin rash, fever, jaundice, nephritis, arthralgia, and edema. Agranulocytosis, which is a very serious reaction and may be fatal, is the most dangerous adverse reaction, but it occurs in less than 1 percent of patients. Patients should be carefully monitored while they are taking this medication because agranulocytosis appears without warning.

449. The answer is D. *(AMA Drug Evaluations Annual 1991, 7/e. p 1953. DiPalma, 3/e. pp 494–495.)* Vitamin D_3 is hydroxylated to 25-OHD_3 (calcifediol). Calcifediol is then hydroxylated in the kidney to the most active form of vitamin D, which is 1,25-$(OH)_2D_3$ (calcitriol). Calcitriol has a rapid onset of action and a short half-life. The administration of calcitriol causes the elevation of serum calcium levels by enhancing the intestinal absorption of calcium. Calcitriol is indicated in vitamin D deficiency, particularly in patients with chronic renal failure or renal tubular disease, hypoparathyroidism, osteomalacia, and rickets. In patients who are treated with a digitalis preparation, it is possible for a drug interaction to occur between digitalis and drugs, such as calcitriol, that can induce hypercalcemia. The elevation of serum calcium levels by calcitriol in the presence of digitalis glycosides can precipitate cardiac arrhythmias.

450. The answer is A. *(Gilman, 8/e. pp 1557–1559.)* Hippocrates recommended beef liver to cure night blindness—a valid suggestion because retinal is necessary to form rhodopsin, the pigment in the eye bleached by light, and liver is a good source of vitamin A (retinol), which can form retinal. In addition to night blindness, vitamin A deficiency can cause keratomalacia, cancellous bone formation, and follicular hyperkeratosis. Follicular hyperkeratosis is one of the early signs of vitamin A deficiency. In cases of hypervitaminosis A, which is due to excessive intake of vitamin A, the signs and symptoms may include fissures of the lips, hyperostosis, hepatomegaly, and severe headache due to elevation of intracranial pressure. The neurologic symptoms caused by the increased intracranial pressure may resemble those of a brain tumor (pseudotumor cerebri).

451. The answer is E. *(DiPalma, 3/e. pp 521–523. Katzung, 4/e. pp 501–503.)* Norethindrone is a 19-nortestosterone derivative. This progestional compound possesses a degree of androgenic and anabolic activity. The major use of norethindrone is as an oral contraceptive, alone or in combination with an estrogen. Some adverse reactions attributed to this progestational agent include increased appetite with weight gain, hirsutism, acne, seborrhea, and cholestatic jaundice. The risk of venous thromboembolic disease is associated with estrogenic agents.

452. The answer is B. *(AMA Drug Evaluations Annual 1991, 7/e. pp 855–858. DiPalma, 3/e. pp 487–488.)* Myxedema coma is a medical emergency and should be treated as soon as the diagnosis is established. Treatment involves the use of several drugs to correct this condition. It appears that the selection of either levothyroxine, liothyronine, or liotrix is appropriate. Levothyroxine, however, is the drug of choice. Supportive treatment of symptoms is also indicated. Maintenance of respiration and administration of fluids and electrolytes, along with glucose if hypoglycemia is diagnosed, should be provided. Since adrenal insufficiency may be present, administration of glucocorticoids is initially recommended. Thyroglobulin, a protein of high molecular weight, is a component of the thyroid gland. Although preparations are available, this drug is not indicated in myxedema coma. Protirelin is a synthetic thyrotropin-stimulating hormone used in the diagnosis of thyroid function. Although lithium was once tested as a drug to treat hyperthyroidism because it induced hypothyroidism, lithium has no place in the therapy of hyperthyroidism. In addition, propylthiouracil is an antithyroid drug used in the management of hyperthyroidism.

453. The answer is E. *(DiPalma, 3/e. pp 523–524. Gilman, 8/e. pp 1403–1407.)* The combination of estrogen and progestin is a more effective means of contraception than is progestin alone. Menstruation will occur with progestin alone, but it may be irregular. Estrogen is thought to cause the increased incidence of thrombophlebitis and cerebral and coronary thrombosis that is found in women taking combined oral contraceptives.

454. This answer is A. *(DiPalma, 3/e. pp 490–492, 494–495. Katzung, 4/e. p 532.)* Parathyroid hormone (PTH) is synthesized by and released from the parathyroid gland; increased synthesis of PTH is a response to low serum calcium concentrations. Resorption and mobilization of calcium and phosphate from bone are increased in response to elevated PTH concentrations. Replacement of body stores of calcium is enhanced by the capacity of PTH to promote increased absorption of calcium by the small intestine in concert with vitamin D, which is the primary factor that enhances intestinal calcium absorption. PTH also causes an increased renal tubular reabsorption of calcium and excretion of phosphate. As a consequence of these effects, the extracellular calcium concentration becomes elevated.

455. The answer is B. *(AMA Drug Evaluations Annual 1991, 7/e. pp 289, 891. DiPalma, 3/e. pp 505–507.)* The oral hypoglycemic agent chlorpropamide is a sulfonylurea compound. The drug is used to treat selected patients with non-insulin-dependent diabetes mellitus (NIDDM, type II). Chlorpropamide has a duration of action of 1 to 3 days. The adverse reaction of hypoglycemia appears to be more common with chlorpropamide than with the other sulfonylurea oral hypoglycemic agents. In addition, water retention and hyponatremia can be caused by chlorpropamide. This adverse reaction is due to an interaction between antidiuretic hormone (ADH) and chlorpropamide. In the collecting duct region of the nephron, chlorpropamide may enhance the effect of antidiuretic hormone and facilitate its release from the posterior pituitary gland. It is reported that chlorpropamide decreases the tolerance to ethanol—an interaction exhibited by flushing of the skin, particularly in the facial area. This disulfiram-like effect is attributed to the inhibition of the oxidation of acetaldehyde that is formed from the biotransformation of ethanol.

456. The answer is C. *(AMA Drug Evaluations Annual 1991, 7/e. pp 965–966. DiPalma, 3/e. pp 520–521.)* Danazol is a 17α-ethinyl testosterone derivative used to treat endometriosis. It appears to be more effective than an estrogen-progestin combination. Since danazol is an androgen derivative, some of the adverse reactions include liver dysfunction, virilism (acne, hirsutism, oily skin, reduced breast size), and reduction in high-density lipoprotein (HDL) cholesterol levels. Other adverse reactions reported for danazol are amenorrhea, weight gain, sweating, vasomotor flushing, and edema. When danazol therapy for endometriosis was compared with the estrogen-progestin regimen, few women discontinued the treatment with danazol because of adverse reactions.

457. The answer is E. *(DiPalma, 3/e. pp 493–494. Gilman, 8/e. pp 1514–1515.)* Enthusiastic overmedication with vitamin D may lead to a toxic syndrome called hypervitaminosis D. The initial symptoms can include weakness, nausea, weight loss, anemia, and mild acidosis. As the excessive doses are continued, signs of nephrotoxicity are manifested, such as polyuria, polydipsia, azotemia, and eventually nephrocalcinosis. In adults osteoporosis can occur. Also there is CNS impairment, which can result in mental retardation and convulsions.

458. The answer is D. *(DiPalma, 3/e. p 544. Katzung, 4/e. pp 485–486.)* The incidence of adverse reactions with administration of methylprednisolone is related to dosage and duration. Psychoses, peptic ulceration with or without hemorrhage, increased susceptibility to infection, edema, osteoporosis, myopathy, and hypokalemic alkalosis can occur. Other adverse reactions include cataracts, hyperglycemia, arrest of growth in children, and iatrogenic Cushing's syndrome. The glucocorticoids are very effective drugs, but they can be very dangerous if not properly administered to a patient.

459. The answer is E. *(AMA Drug Evaluations Annual 1991, 7/e. pp 887–892. DiPalma, 3/e. pp 504–507.)* Glyburide is classified as a second-generation oral hypoglycemic agent. It causes hypoglycemia by stimulating the release of insulin from the pancreas and increases peripheral sensitivity to insulin. The drug is well absorbed upon oral administration and is biotransformed by the liver. Its duration of action is about 12 to 24 h, whereas the duration of action of chlorpropamide is 1 to 3 days. Glyburide has a mild course of action, whereas chlorpropamide can cause water retention and dilutional hyponatremia. In addition chlorpropamide may decrease tolerance to ethanol in that ethanol in the presence of chlorpropamide causes flushing of the skin, particularly in the facial area. Glyburide has not been reported to cause this effect when ethanol is consumed.

460. The answer is B. *(DiPalma, 3/e. pp 414, 504–505, 540. Gilman, 8/e. pp 1438–1440, 1484–1485.)* The concurrent administration of hydrocortisone and an oral hypoglycemic agent, such as chlorpropamide, reduces the effectiveness of the hypoglycemic agent in controlling blood glucose levels in patients who have non-insulin-dependent diabetes mellitus. Hydrocortisone and prednisone induce hyperglycemia by enhancing gluconeogenesis in the liver and periphery. In addition the steroids also promote the release of glucagon from the cells of the pancreas to eventually increase blood glucose levels. Hydrocortisone possesses significant mineralocorticoid activity in addition to its glucocorticoid effect. The mineralocorticoid action of hydrocortisone alters electrolyte metabolism. Hydrocortisone enhances the retention of sodium and water in the body and augments the secretion of potassium, which can lead to hypokalemia. Prednisone also possesses a degree of mineralocorticoid activity and may produce hypokalemia. The diuretics hydrochlorothiazide and bumetanide can cause hypokalemia. In addition these diuretics cause hyperglycemia by inhibiting the release of insulin from the pancreas. If patients are to receive hydrocortisone and a loop or a thiazide diuretic, their potassium levels should be monitored to prevent potassium depletion.

461–464. The answers are: 461-A, 462-B, 463-E, 464-D. *(AMA Drug Evaluations Annual 1991, 7/e. pp 668, 844, 846, 848, 995, 1794. DiPalma, 3/e. pp 515, 527, 544.)* Ethinyl estradiol is a synthetic estrogen that is not readily biotransformed by the liver. This estrogen derivative is used as a "morning-after" contraceptive when it is given orally, in very large doses, within 24 to 48 h after sexual intercourse. Diethylstilbestrol, a nonsteroidal estrogen, is also used as a "morning-after" contraceptive.

Spironolactone is a competitive inhibitor of the mineralocorticoid aldosterone. Aldosterone acts in the collecting duct of the nephron unit to promote the reabsorption of sodium and the excretion of potassium. In the condition of primary hyperaldosteronism caused by adrenal adenoma, spironolactone is used prior to surgery to decrease urinary excretion of potassium. The drug is indicated in the prolonged treatment of hyperaldosteronism caused by hyperplasia of both adrenal glands. Spironolactone is also used as a potassium-sparing diuretic in the treatment of edema and essential hypertension—generally in combination with another diuretic agent.

Leuprolide is a peptide that is related to gonadotropin-releasing hormone or luteinizing hormone–releasing hormone. This agent is used to treat metastatic prostate carcinoma. A hypogonadal state is produced in the patient from the continuous administration of leuprolide. Testosterone levels in the body become significantly reduced.

Fludrocortisone is a synthetic steroid compound that exhibits profound mineralocorticoid activity and some glucocorticoid activity. Electrolyte and water metabolisms are affected by the administration of this compound. Fludrocortisone promotes the reabsorption of sodium and the urinary excretion of potassium and hydrogen ions in the collecting duct of the nephron. The drug is indicated for mineralocorticoid replacement therapy in primary adrenal insufficiency.

Steroid synthesis in the adrenal cortex is inhibited by the administration of aminoglutethimide. The formation of pregnenolone from cholesterol is reduced and as a consequence of this action the secretion from the gland of steroids, such as cortisol and aldosterone, is decreased. Aminoglutethimide is indicated in Cushing's syndrome to reduce the release of cortisol.

465–468. The answers are: 465-A, 466-B, 467-B, 468-E. *(DiPalma, 3/e. pp 483, 484, 488, 489. Gilman, 8/e. pp 1363, 1371, 1373, 1377, 1379.)* Agents that can interfere directly or indirectly with the synthesis of thyroid hormone are called *thyroid inhibitors*. Thiocyanate, an ionic inhibitor, interferes with the ability of the thyroid to concentrate iodide by acting as a competitive inhibitor. Thiocyanate and other ionic inhibitors, such as perchlorate, nitrate, and fluoborate, are hydrated monovalent anions having a size similar to that of iodide.

Methimazole (Tapazole), together with propylthiouracil, is classified as an antithyroid drug that interferes directly with thyroid hormone synthesis. Antithyroid drugs interfere with the oxidation and incorporation of iodide into organic form and inhibit the formation of iodothyronines from the peroxidase-mediated coupling of iodotyrosines. These drugs may act by binding to peroxidase, by interacting with substrates, or by interfering with the production of hydrogen peroxide, which (in addition to oxygen) is a biologic oxidant required for the synthesis of thyroid hormones.

Iodide, most ancient of therapeutic agents for thyroid disorders, inhibits the secretion of thyroid hormone by retarding both the pinocytosis of colloid and proteolysis. This effect is observed in euthyroid as well as hyperthyroid persons.

Triiodothyronine is not classified as a thyroid inhibitor; it is an amino acid derivative of thyronine and results from the oxidative coupling of monoiodotyrosyl and diiodotyrosyl residues.

^{131}I, the most often used radioisotope of iodine, is rapidly absorbed by the thyroid and is deposited in follicular colloid. From the site of its deposition, ^{131}I causes fibrosis of the thyroid subsequent to pyknosis and necrosis of the follicular cells.

469–471. The answers are: 469-J, 470-D, 471-E. *(DiPalma, 3/e. pp 434–435, 484–488, 493–495. Gilman, 8/e. pp 1438, 1484, 1490.)* Propylthiouracil and methimazole are classified as thioamides that are used in the long-term treatment of hyperthyroidism. These drugs are reducing agents that inhibit the enzymatic oxidation of iodide ion to active iodine and reduce the coupling reaction of iodotyrosines in the thyroid gland. Both of these reactions are mediated by peroxidase. In addition, propylthiouracil prevents the peripheral conversion of T_4 to T_3. Other drugs such as glucocorticoids, propranolol, and amiodarone also interfere with the cellular conversion of T_4 to T_3.

Diazoxide is a thiazide derivative used intravenously in the treatment of acute hypertensive crisis. Although this compound is a thiazide, it promotes the retention of sodium and water on chronic administration. In a manner similar to that of the thiazide diuretics, diazoxide can produce hyperglycemia by inhibition of insulin secretion. Diazoxide may also have some ability to inhibit peripheral glucose utilization and to stimulate gluconeogenesis. Advantage is taken of the hyperglycemic action of diazide in that it is used orally in the treatment of various types of hypoglycemia. Drugs such as acetohexamide, chlorpropamide, and glyburide cause the stimulation of beta cells in the pancreas to promote the secretion of insulin.

The only agent from the list of drugs in this question that inhibits bone resorption is etidronate. It prevents hypoxyapatite crystal formation, growth, and dissolution. Sodium etidronate is used in the therapy of Paget's disease.

472–474. The answers are: 472-G, 473-E, 474-L. *(AMA Drug Evaluations Annual 1991, 7/e. pp 942–943. DiPalma, 3/e. pp 502, 512.)* Ethinyl estradiol is a synthetic estrogen derivative that is orally effective. It is used in combination with progestins as an oral contraceptive. Ethinyl estradiol is also used alone in various gynecologic disorders such as menopausal symptoms, breast cancer in selected postmenopausal women, and prostatic carcinoma. A major adverse reaction with ethinyl estradiol and other estrogens involves the coagulation reaction. Estrogens increase the synthesis of vitamin K–dependent factors II, VII, IX, and X. The effect on the coagulation scheme can alter the prothrombin time of persons who are using oral anticoagulants (e.g., warfarin). In addition, estrogens can increase the incidence of thromboembolic disorders through their procoagulation effect.

In the therapy of diabetes mellitus the effectiveness of insulin to regulate glucose levels in the body can be reduced by simultaneous administration of other drugs. Glucose levels in the body are elevated by the administration of glucocorticoid (e.g., hydrocortisone), dextrothyroxine, epinephrine, thiazide diuretics (e.g., hydrochlorothiazide), and levothyroxine. The drug-induced hyperglycemia counteracts the hypoglycemic action of insulin preparations. In addition, any drug that induces hyperglycemia can also reduce the effectiveness of the oral hypoglycemic agents such as tolbutamide, acetohexamide, and glyburide.

Spironolactone is classified as a potassium-sparing diuretic. Spironolactone is a competitive inhibitor of aldosterone. It has a mild diuretic effect but is generally used with other diuretics such as thiazides or loop diuretics to prevent the development of hypokalemia. The drug is also used in endocrinology in the diagnosis and treatment of hyperaldosteronism. Another therapeutic use of spironolactone is in the treatment of hirsutism in females, whether it is idiopathic or related to excessive androgen secretion. The drug causes a decrease in the rate of growth and the density of facial hair, possibly through inhibition of excessive androgen production and an effect on the hair follicle.

Toxicology

- Air Pollutants
  - Benzene
  - Carbon monoxide
  - Carbon tetrachloride
  - Chloroform
  - Nitrogen dioxide
  - Ozone
  - Sulfur dioxide
  - Tetrachloroethylene
  - Toluene
  - 1,1,1-Trichloroethane
  - Trichloroethylene
- Heavy Metals
  - Aluminum
  - Arsenic
  - Cadmium
  - Iron
  - Lead
  - Mercury
  - Zinc
- Heavy Metal Antagonists
  - Calcium disodium edetate
  - Deferoxamine
  - Dimercaprol
  - Penicillamine
- Herbicide
  - 2,4-Dichlorophenoxyacetic acid
- Organophosphorus Insecticides
  - Diazinon
  - Malathion
  - Parathion
  - Antidotes: atropine and pralidoxime
- Toxic Gas
  - Carbon monoxide
- Toxic Ion
  - Cyanide

DIRECTIONS: Each question below contains five suggested responses. Select the **one best** response to each question.

475. All the following statements regarding drug interactions are true EXCEPT

(A) aspirin may increase the hypoprothrombinemic effect of dicumarol
(B) combining amphetamine and levothyroxine may cause cardiac tachyarrhythmias
(C) amitriptyline may increase the sedative effect of ethanol
(D) cholestyramine enhances the hepatotoxicity of acetaminophen
(E) benztropine would increase the risk of urinary retention, paralytic ileus, and blurred vision associated with thioridazine

476. Convulsions caused by drug poisoning are most commonly associated with

(A) phenobarbital
(B) diazepam
(C) strychnine
(D) chlorpromazine
(E) phenytoin

477. Alkalinization of the urine with sodium bicarbonate is useful in the treatment of poisoning with

(A) aspirin (acetylsalicylic acid)
(B) amphetamine
(C) morphine
(D) phencyclidine
(E) cocaine

478. All the following statements are true about arsenic poisoning EXCEPT

(A) acute poisoning causes severe diarrhea and difficulty swallowing
(B) signs of chronic poisoning include peripheral neuritis, hypotension, and anemia
(C) death following acute intoxication may be due to hypovolemic shock
(D) dimercaprol is the primary agent used in the treatment of chronic arsenic poisoning
(E) gingivitis, stomatitis, and salivation can occur

479. Which of the following is an agent useful in the treatment of severe poisoning by organophosphorus insecticides, such as parathion?

(A) Ethylenediaminetetraacetic acid (EDTA)
(B) Pralidoxime (2-PAM)
(C) *N*-Acetylcysteine
(D) Carbachol
(E) Diethyldithiocarbamic acid

480. All the following are true of cyanide poisoning EXCEPT

(A) it causes convulsions and coma
(B) it produces bright red venous blood
(C) it produces ECG abnormalities and bradycardia
(D) it is treated with sodium thiocyanate
(E) it is treated with sodium nitrite

481. Activated charcoal may be used to treat poisoning by all the following drugs EXCEPT

(A) phenobarbital
(B) carbamazepine (Tegretol)
(C) proxyphene (Darvon)
(D) methanol
(E) aspirin

482. All the following statements are true for methanol intoxication EXCEPT

(A) blurred vision and hyperemia of the optic disc may develop
(B) it may produce bradycardia, coma, and seizures
(C) treatment includes administration of ethanol
(D) ascorbic acid corrects the metabolic alkalosis
(E) treatment may include hemodialysis

483. *N*-Acetylbenzoquinoneimine is the hepatotoxic metabolite of which drug?

(A) Sulindac (Clinoril)
(B) Acetaminophen
(C) Isoniazid
(D) Indomethacin (Indocin)
(E) Procainamide

484. All the following drugs may produce a syndrome of flushing, headache, nausea, vomiting, sweating, hypotension, and confusion after ethanol consumption EXCEPT

(A) amitriptyline (Elavil)
(B) cefoperazine (Cefobid)
(C) acetohexamide (Dymelor)
(D) moxalactam (Moxane)
(E) disulfiram (Antabuse)

485. All the following statements are true for carbon monoxide EXCEPT

(A) poisoning is effectively treated with 100% oxygen
(B) it binds to hemoglobin, reducing the oxygen-carrying capacity of blood
(C) carboxyhemoglobin levels below 15 percent rarely produce symptoms
(D) symptoms of poisoning include headache, convulsions, and respiratory and cardiovascular depression
(E) it inhibits ferricytochrome oxidase

486. Rapid intravenous administration of this drug causes hypocalcemic tetany.

(A) Dimercaprol
(B) Edetate disodium
(C) Deferoxamine
(D) Penicillamine
(E) *N*-Acetylcysteine

487. Acute intermittent porphyria is a contraindication to the use of

(A) enflurane (Ethrane)
(B) nitrous oxide
(C) ketamine (Ketalar)
(D) diazepam (Valium)
(E) thiopental sodium

488. All the following drugs can cause hepatic toxicity EXCEPT

(A) valproic acid (Depakene)
(B) halothane (Fluothane)
(C) thiopental sodium
(D) enflurane (Ethrane)
(E) ethanol

DIRECTIONS: Each group of questions below consists of lettered headings followed by a set of numbered items. For each numbered item select the **one** lettered heading with which it is **most** closely associated. Each lettered heading may be used **once, more than once, or not at all.**

Questions 489–491

Many drugs when given to a pregnant woman produce significant adverse effects on the fetus. For each of the drugs below, match the most likely adverse effect.

(A) Vaginal adenocarcinoma
(B) Congenital goiter, hypothyroidism
(C) Masculinization of female fetus
(D) Gray baby syndrome
(E) Prolonged neonatal hypoglycemia

489. Diethylstilbestrol

490. Chlorpropamide

491. Methimazole

Questions 492–494

For each of the agents below, select the specific antidote.

(A) Leucovorin
(B) Naloxone (Narcan)
(C) Physostigmine
(D) Ethanol
(E) Diazepam (Valium)

492. Atropine

493. Heroin

494. Methotrexate

Questions 495–497

For each of the agents below taken by a nursing mother, select the potential toxicity to the neonate.

(A) Pyridoxine deficiency
(B) Kernicterus
(C) Suppression of thyroid function
(D) Staining of developing teeth
(E) Sedation

495. Sulfonamides

496. Tetracycline

497. Propylthiouracil

Questions 498–500

For each patient, select the drug or agent most likely to cause the toxic effect.

(A) Aluminum
(B) Bismuth
(C) Carbon monoxide
(D) Dapsone
(E) Methanol
(F) Gentamicin
(G) Lead
(H) Metronidazole
(I) Nalidixic acid
(J) Primaquine
(K) Ethylene glycol
(L) Sulfamethoxazole
(M) Sulfasalazine
(N) Tetracycline

498. A 49-year-old woman is treated for an *E. coli* urinary tract infection. During treatment the woman experiences hemolysis

499. A 3-year-old boy consumed a liquid from a container in the family garage. He shows central nervous system depression, acidosis, suppressed respiration, and oxalate crystals in the urine. Beside supportive and corrective measures, ethanol was administered to the child

500. A 4-year-old girl has the following signs and symptoms: ataxia; tremors; constipation; weakness of extensor muscles; colic; increased δ-aminolevulinic aciduria; and basophilic, stippled erythroblasts

Toxicology

Answers

475. The answer is D. *(DiPalma, 3/e. p 274. Katzung, 4/e. pp 831–835.)* Drug interactions may be beneficial or more often may lead to increased incidences of adverse or toxic effects. Aspirin and other salicylates may increase the hypoprothrombinemic effect of dicumarol. This is because aspirin inhibits platelet aggregation, has a hypoprothrombinemic effect, and displaces dicumarol from plasma proteins. Amphetamines should not be combined with thyroid hormones (e.g., levothyroxine) for weight reduction since the combination can lead to palpitations, increased heart rate, and even cardiac tachyarrhythmias. Cholestyramine would not enhance the effects of acetaminophen. Cholestyramine reduces the oral absorption of acetaminophen and several other drugs, and this reduces the plasma concentrations. Benztropine, a muscarinic blocking agent used in the treatment of parkinsonism, would increase the risk of anticholinergic adverse effects associated with phenothiazines (e.g., thioridazine). Amitriptyline possesses a sedative effect. In combination with ethanol, amitriptyline enhances the central depressant properties of ethanol.

476. The answer is C. *(Gilman, 8/e. pp 1632–1633. Katzung, 4/e. p 257.)* Strychnine acts as a competitive antagonist of glycine, the predominant postsynaptic inhibitory transmitter in the brain and spinal cord. The fatal adult dose is 50 to 100 mg. Persons poisoned by strychnine suffer convulsions that progress to full tetanic convulsions. Because the diaphragm and thoracic muscles are fully contracted, the patient cannot breathe. Hypoxia eventually causes medullary paralysis and death. Control of the convulsions and respiratory support are the immediate objectives of therapy. Diazepam may be preferred to a barbiturate in controlling the convulsions because it offers less concomitant respiratory depression. Poisoning caused by the other drugs listed in the question is not associated with convulsions but with depression of the central nervous system.

477. The answer is A. *(DiPalma, 3/e. p 42. Gilman, 8/e. pp 18–20.)* Sodium bicarbonate is excreted principally in the urine and alkalinizes it. Increasing urinary pH interferes with the passive renal tubular reabsorption of organic acids (such as aspirin and phenobarbital) by increasing the ionic form of the drug in the tubular filtrate. This would increase their excretion. Excretion of organic bases (such as amphetamine, cocaine, phencyclidine, and morphine) would be enhanced by acidifying the urine.

478. The answer is E. *(DiPalma, 3/e. pp 688–691.)* Arsenic is an active constituent of fungicides, herbicides, and pesticides. Symptoms of acute toxicity include tightness in the throat, difficulty in swallowing, and stomach pains. Projectile vomiting and severe diarrhea can lead to hypovolemic shock and death. Chronic poisoning may cause peripheral neuritis, anemia, skin keratosis, and capillary dilation leading to hypotension. Dimercaprol is the primary agent used in the treatment of arsenic poisoning. Gingivitis, stomatitis, and salivation are symptoms associated with acute mercury poisoning.

479. The answer is B. *(DiPalma, 3/e. pp 142–143, 238, 320. Gilman, 8/e. p 122. Katzung, 4/e. pp 76, 77, 81.)* The organophosphorus insecticides inactivate cholinesterases, which results in accumulation of endogenous acetylcholine in nerve tissue and effector organs. Very severe cases of acute poisoning should be treated first with atropine followed immediately by intravenous pralidoxime (2-PAM). Atropine inhibits the actions of acetylcholine at muscarinic cholinergic receptors, whereas 2-PAM reactivates the inactivated cholinesterases. The effectiveness of 2-PAM in reversing cholinesterase inhibition depends upon early treatment inasmuch as the "aged" inhibited enzyme cannot be reactivated. Diethyldithiocarbamic acid is the active biotransformation product of disulfiram, which is an irreversible inhibitor of aldehyde dehydrogenase. *N*-Acetylcysteine is an antidote used in the treatment of acetaminophen overdosage to prevent hepatotoxicities. Carbachol is a cholinomimetic drug and ethylenediaminetetraacetic acid (EDTA) is a chelating agent. These compounds have no therapeutic value in the treatment of organophosphate poisoning.

480. The answer is D. *(DiPalma, 3/e. pp 702–705. Gilman, 8/e. pp 1630–1631.)* Cyanide can produce cytotoxic hypoxia. It is eliminated chiefly in the form of thiocyanate ion, but this pathway is limited by the endogenous supply of thiosulfate. In cyanide poisoning, symptoms may include salivation, nausea, anxiety, convulsions, vertigo, cardiac arrhythmias, bradycardia, and a transient respiratory stimulation followed by respiratory failure. In addition, venous blood becomes a bright red, since the erythrocytes are highly saturated with oxygen. The administration of sodium nitrite forms methemoglobin that competes with cytochrome oxidase for the cyanide ion, thus protecting cytochrome oxidase. After sodium nitrite infusion, sodium thiosulfate (not sodium thiocyanate) should be infused slowly over a period of 10 min to accelerate detoxification. Amyl nitrite administered by inhalation may also be useful.

481. The answer is D. *(Gilman, 8/e. p 58. Katzung, 4/e. pp 284–285, 756–757.)* Activated charcoal, a fine, black powder with a high adsorptive capacity, is considered to be a highly valuable agent in the treatment of many kinds of drug poisoning. Drugs that are well adsorbed by activated charcoal include primaquine, propoxyphene, dextroamphetamine, chlorpheniramine, phenobarbital, carbamazepine, digoxin, and aspirin. Mineral acids, alkalines, tolbutamide, and other drugs that are insoluble in acidic aqueous solution are not well adsorbed. Charcoal also does not bind cyanide, lithium, iron, or alcohols.

482. The answer is D. *(DiPalma, 3/e. pp 238–239. Gilman, 8/e. p 624.)* Acute intoxication with methanol is common in chronic alcoholics. Headache, vertigo, vomiting, abdominal pain, dyspnea, blurred vision, and hyperemia of the optic disc can occur. Visual disturbances are caused by damage of retinal cells and the optic nerve by methanol metabolites. Severe cases of intoxication can lead to blindness. Other symptoms include bradycardia, prolonged coma, seizures, acidosis, and death by respiratory depression. Since methanol is biotransformed by alcohol dehydrogenase to highly toxic products (formaldehyde and formic acid), ethanol, which has high affinity for the enzyme, is useful in therapy because it reduces the biotransformation of methanol. Other treatments include hemodialysis to enhance removal of methanol and its products and alkalinization to reverse metabolic acidosis. 4-Methylprazole, an inhibitor of alcohol dehydrogenase, has also been proposed for treatment.

483. The answer is B. *(DiPalma, 3/e. pp 317, 320, 375, 626. Gilman, 8/e. pp 657–658, 852.)* Hepatic necrosis can occur with overdosage of acetaminophen. The hepatic toxicity is the result of the biotransformation of acetaminophen to *N*-acetylbenzoquinoneimine, which reacts with hepatic proteins and glutathione. This metabolite depletes glutathione stores and produces necrosis. The administration of *N*-acetylcysteine restores hepatic concentrations of glutathione and reduces the potential hepatotoxicity. Sulindac is biotransformed to sulindac sulfide, the active form of the drug. Both sulindac and its metabolites are excreted in the urine and in the feces. Indomethacin undergoes a demethylation reaction and an *N*-deacylation reaction. The parent compound and its metabolites are mainly excreted in the urine. Procainamide is converted to an active metabolite by an acetylation reaction. The product that is formed is *N*-acetylprocainamide (NAPA). In addition, procainamide is hydrolyzed by amidases. An *N*-acetylation reaction occurs also in the biotransformation of isoniazid. In the liver the enzyme *N*-acetyl transferase converts isoniazid to acetyl-isoniazid.

484. The answer is A. *(DiPalma, 3/e. pp 237–238.)* Disulfiram is a pharmacologic adjunct in the treatment of alcoholism. When given to a person who has consumed ethanol, it produces flushing, headache, nausea, vomiting, sweating, hypotension, and confusion. The mechanism involves inhibition of aldehyde dehydrogenase; thus acetaldehyde accumulates as a result of ethanol metabolism. Many other agents produce disulfiram-like reactions when administered with ethanol, though their mechanisms have not been established; these include cephalosporins (cefoperazine, cefoperazone, moxalactam), phentolamine, metronidazole, and the sulfonylureas (e.g., acetohexamide and tolbutamide). The tricyclic antidepressant amitriptyline causes sedation. The interaction between ethanol and amitriptyline produces an enhancement of the central depressant properties of ethanol.

485. The answer is E. *(DiPalma, 3/e. pp 700–702. Katzung, 4/e. p 735.)* Carbon monoxide is a common cause of accidental and suicidal poisoning. Its affinity for hemoglobin is 250 times greater than that of oxygen. It therefore binds to hemoglobin and reduces the oxygen-carrying capacity of blood. The symptoms of poisoning are due to tissue hypoxia and progress from headache and fatigue to confusion, syncope, tachycardia, coma, convulsions, shock, respiratory depression, and cardiovascular collapse. Carboxyhemoglobin levels below 15 percent rarely produce symptoms; above 40 percent symptoms become severe. Treatment includes establishment of an airway, supportive therapy, and administration of 100% oxygen. It is the cyanide ion that binds to ferricytochrome oxidase and impairs cellular oxygen use, which leads to histotoxic hypoxia.

486. The answer is B. *(DiPalma, 3/e. pp 320, 455–456, 692–695. Gilman, 8/e. pp 1607–1612.)* The chelation agent edetate disodium (Na_2EDTA) causes hypocalcemic tetany on rapid intravenous administration. This effect of edetate disodium is not observed on slow infusion (15 mg/min) since extracirculatory stores are available to prevent a significant reduction in plasma calcium levels. When edetate calcium disodium is given intravenously, hypocalcemia does not develop even when large doses are required. Edetate calcium disodium is used in the diagnosis and treatment of lead intoxication. Edetate disodium is used to treat acute hypercalcemia. The other drugs listed do not cause hypocalcemia. Dimercaprol (BAL) forms chelation complexes between its sulfhydryl groups and metals and is used in the treatment of arsenic and mercury poisoning as well as in certain cases of lead poisoning in children. Penicillamine is the drug of choice in treating Wilson's disease. The agent is also used in the therapy of copper, mercury, and lead poisoning. *N*-Acetylcysteine is an antidote used in the treatment of overdosage with acetaminophen to prevent hepatoxicity.

487. The answer is E. *(DiPalma, 3/e. p 215. Gilman, 8/e. pp 301–305.)* Induction of anesthesia by parenteral administration of thiopental sodium (Pentothal) and other barbiturates is absolutely contraindicated in patients who have acute intermittent porphyria. These patients have a defect in regulation of δ-aminolevulinic acid synthetase; thus, administration of a barbiturate that increases this enzyme may cause a dangerous increase in levels of porphyrins. Administration of a barbiturate would exacerbate the symptoms of gastrointestinal and neurologic disturbances, cause extensive demyelination of peripheral and cranial nerves, and could lead to death.

488. The answer is C. *(DiPalma, 3/e. pp 200–202, 235, 286. Gilman, 8/e. pp 286–294, 450–452.)* Halothane and enflurane are effective general anesthetics; however, along with other halogenated compounds such as chloroform and carbon tetrachloride, they share a propensity to cause hepatotoxicity. Hepatic function is impaired during treatment with halothane and enflurane, but this is rapidly reversible upon termination of treatment. Hepatic necrosis may result from biotransformation of halothane and enflurane to reactive intermediates that react with liver macromolecules. Chronic abuse of ethanol can cause alcoholic hepatitis and cirrhosis of the liver. The use of valproic acid in epilepsy can produce abnormal effects on hepatic function, and although it is rare, hepatitis can occur.

489–491. The answers are: 489-A, 490-E, 491-B. *(Katzung, 4/e. p 764.)* There are many drugs that can produce significant adverse effects on the fetus when given to a pregnant woman. Among these are diethylstilbestrol, which has been shown to produce vaginal adenocarcinoma in female offspring. The incidence of clear-cell vaginal and cervical adenocarcinoma in women exposed to estrogens in utero has been estimated at 0.01 to 0.1 percent. Methimazole may cause hypothyroidism and congenital goiter by reducing thyroid hormone synthesis. Testosterone and derivatives can produce masculinization of the female fetus. Owing to low levels of glucuronyl transferase in the fetus, chloramphenicol increases the risk of gray baby syndrome. Sulfonylurea derivatives, e.g., chlorpropamide, can cause prolonged hypoglycemia in the neonate by stimulating excessive insulin secretion.

492–494. The answers are: 492-C, 493-B, 494-A. *(Katzung, 4/e. p 759.)* The peripheral and central nervous system effects of atropine poisoning may be reversed with physostigmine. Because physostigmine is biotransformed more rapidly than atropine, repeated doses may be necessary. Neostigmine and other quaternary anticholinesterase drugs that do not cross the blood-brain barrier cannot be used to treat the central nervous system effects of atropine.

Naloxone is a competitive antagonist at opioid receptors and is therefore useful in treating overdose with opioid drugs (e.g., morphine, heroin). Because of its short duration of action, repeated doses are usually necessary.

Methotrexate inhibits dihydrofolate reductase and limits the supply of N^5-formyltetrahydrofolate, which is required in the synthesis of thymidylate. Leucovorin (citrovorum factor of N^5-formyltetrahydrofolate) can reduce the toxic effects of methotrexate. Methotrexate therapy followed by leucovorin is a chemotherapeutic regimen for some neoplastic disorders.

495–497. The answers are: 495-B, 496-D, 497-C. *(DiPalma, 3/e. p 489. Katzung, 4/e. pp 767–768.)* Many drugs taken by nursing mothers can be detected in breast milk. Though some agents (e.g., ampicillin, acetaminophen) have minimal effects, many agents prove to be potentially dangerous.

Sulfonamides have been found in breast milk of nursing mothers. The compounds are highly protein-bound and thus compete with bilirubin for binding to plasma albumin. The higher levels of free bilirubin increase the risk of kernicterus.

Tetracyclines concentrate in breast milk and may cause permanent tooth staining in the infant by binding to calcium. From midpregnancy to 4 to 6 months after birth is the period of greatest danger for deciduous anterior teeth. From 6 months to 5 years of age is the most dangerous period for the permanent anterior teeth.

Propylthiouracil, an agent useful in treatment of hyperthyroidism, can concentrate in breast milk of nursing mothers. The drug significantly suppresses thyroid function in the infant.

Isoniazid reaches rapid equilibrium between breast milk and maternal blood. It can cause pyridoxine deficiency if the mother or child does not receive supplementation.

Central nervous system depressants, such as diazepam or barbiturates, can cause significant sedation in nursing infants.

498–500. The answers are: 498-L, 499-K, 500-G. *(DiPalma, 3/e. pp 239, 623–626, 632, 653–656, 683–687. Gilman, 8/e. pp 1052, 1055–1056, 1159–1160, 1593–1598.)* Sulfonamides can cause acute hemolytic anemia. In some patients it may be related to a sensitization phenomenon and in other patients the hemolysis is due to a glucose-6-phosphate dehydrogenase deficiency. Sulfamethoxazole alone or in combination with trimethoprim is used to treat urinary tract infections. The sulfonamide sulfasalazine is employed in the treatment of ulcerative colitis. Dapsone, a drug used in the treatment of leprosy, and primaquine, an antimalarial agent, can produce hemolysis, particularly in patients with a glucose-6-phosphate dehydrogenase deficiency.

Ethylene glycol, an industrial solvent and an antifreeze compound, is involved in accidental and intentional poisonings. This compound is initially oxidized by alcohol dehydrogenase and then further biotransformed to oxalic acid and other products. Oxalate crystals are found in various tissues of the body and are excreted by the kidney. Deposition of oxalate crystals in the kidney causes renal toxicity. Ethylene glycol is also a central nervous system depressant. In cases of ethylene glycol poisoning, ethanol is administered to reduce the first step in the biotransformation of ethylene glycol and, thereby, prevent the formation of oxalate and other products.

Lead poisoning in children is most often caused by the ingestion of paint chips that contain lead. Older housing units and homes were painted with lead compounds that produced various colors. Chronic lead intoxication causes such symptoms as basophilic stippling, increased δ-aminolevulinic aciduria, tremors, weakness of extensor muscles, constipation, lead line, and colic.

Bibliography

AMA Drug Evaluations Annual 1991, 7/e. American Medical Association, Chicago, 1986.

DiPalma JR, DiGregorio GJ: *Basic Pharmacology in Medicine,* 3/e. New York, McGraw-Hill, 1990.

Gilman AG, et al (eds): *The Pharmacological Basis of Therapeutics,* 8/e. New York, Macmillan, 1990.

Katzung BG: *Basic and Clinical Pharmacology,* 4/e. East Norwalk, CT, Appleton & Lange, 1989.

Wilson JD, et al (eds): *Harrison's Principles of Internal Medicine,* 12/e. New York, McGraw-Hill, 1991.